"Look at yourself. You are disgusting. Your wife will get off the plane from Germany with your baby, look at you, and get back on the plane and go home."

Jerry's fingers wrapped around the psychologist's ashtray and his knuckles shone white with the ferocity of his grip. He dared not strike back at the inhumanity of the man's comment. This man held a sway over his life that was greater than his own . . . .

AF698191

Power To Live Through Nutrition

By JAMES W. McAFEE
Director of Nutritional Research
Image Awareness Corp.

PUBLISHED BY IMAGE AWARENESS CORP.

P.O. BOX 3307
AUBURN, CA 95604

Publisher's note: This book offers general nutritional guidelines toward physical and mental well-being; the reader is advised to consult his personal physician for specific application of dietary principles or fasting to best fit individual needs and remedy specific ailments.

Library of Congress Catalogue Card Number 80-82331. ISBN 0-9604592-0-0, paper. Copyright ©1980 by James W. McAfee. All rights reserved. Printed in the United States of America.

Photo credits: Photos from Weston Price's classic book, *Nutrition and Physical Degeneration,* and Francis Pottenger's cat studies are used with permission of the Price-Pottenger Nutrition Foundation, P.O. Box 2614, La Mesa, California 92041.

The line drawings are used with permission of the Neo-Life Company of America. The rat photographs were supplied by Donald E. Pickett.

Published by the "Image" Awareness Corporation, P.O. Box 3307, Auburn, California 95604.

ACKNOWLEDGMENTS

I owe a debt of gratitude to the great nutritional pioneers of the past who opened the door to our understanding of how diet affects health. Among these men and women are Weston A. Price, D.D.S., Dr. Francis M. Pottenger, Jr., and Adele Davis.

Contemporary men and women who deserve special recognition include Nathan Pritikin, Linda Clark, Covert Bailey, Dr. Carlton Fredericks, Dr. Emmanuel Cheraskin, Dr. Marshall Ringsdorf, Dr. Elizabeth Rees, Dr. Hans Selye, and Dr. Rudolph Alsleben. The work of Dr. Charles McGee has been a special inspiration.

I feel a great debt of gratitude to the many psychologists and psychiatrists who are warm and loving human beings. We as a society owe a special debt to those who have taught us the relationship between mental health and nutrition. Among their number are Jay Adams, Dr. Michael Lesser, Dr. Richard Kunin, Dr. Abram Hoffer, Dr. Carl Pfeiffer, Dr. Linus Pauling, Alex Schauss, Dr. Roger Williams, Dr. Theron Randolph and Dr. William Philpott.

There are many more who deserve to be mentioned and I beg their indulgence for the omission. Their names would fill a book.

A special word of gratitude to Pat Brooks who helped formulate the idea for the organization of this book.

NOTE

The mental hospital in which I worked and one of the physicians who worked with Jerry were later investigated by governmental agencies and publically criticized in the media. They were not exemplary of the best their professions have to offer.

This book is dedicated to Pat Odneal who spent her life making people aware of the benefits of good nutrition and who suffered a tragic death and to Jerry whose story had to be told.

AUTHOR'S PREFACE

Carol (not her real name) sat rigidly in the soft leather chair in front of me. Her eyes were large behind her glasses. Someone in the group had just told her that they were feeling much better after supplementing their diet. Carol said, "Can't I get all the nutrition I need from the food I eat?" She directed her narrow face and Roman nose toward me and her eyes widened as she said, "Couldn't food supplements become addicting?"

Under other circumstances I might have pointed out that it is difficult to get the nutrients we need from our food due to conditions of growing, transport, processing and cooking. As I looked at her, however, a new thought entered my mind. I said, "What do you really want out of life? Do you merely want the energy to stand upright or do you want to be a dynamo charged with energy? Most people make the mistake of thinking that nutrition is an all or nothing affair, but it is not."

The nutritional provision of nature is rarely, if ever, completely adequate. Dr. Roger Williams points out that a cake of yeast given a perfect environment would become a huge ball within one week. Obviously, yeast rarely has a perfect environment.

Nutrition is frequently submarginal in people as well. I will never forget the study reported by Dr. Cheraskin in which he described how he punctured the gum of his dental students with a probe then observed the healing time with varying amounts of vitamin C in the diet. He found that the more vitamin C his subjects were given the more rapidly the healing occured. He humorously concluded his report by saying that he was forced to end the study because he feared the gum would heal before he could get the probe out.

The significant point to be noted about this work is that a small amount of vitamin C was adequate for healing, but a larger amount of the nutrient enabled the body to operate on a higher level of efficiency than would otherwise have been possible. Similar results were reported with zinc, an essential mineral.

It is my contention that nutrition is not an all or nothing affair, but a matter of degree. The more adequate our nutrition, the more efficiently our bodies operate. The difference between passable health and vibrant health for many people could very easily be small changes in the diet and simple supplementation of their diet with the nutrients essential for health.

To show how small a change can have an effect upon the body, Linus Pauling reports an experiment where the simple addition of orange juice to the diets of school children increased their IQ scores 3.6 points. He felt the change was due to additional vitamin C in the diet. *(Vitamin C and the Common Cold.)* In one study of children on poor versus good diets, investigators found a difference in IQ scores of 22.6 points.

As Carol heard some of these thoughts she became quite excited. She realized that the true function of good diet is not to cure disease but to enable us to live our lives with undiminished potential.

Because good nutrition is not an all or nothing affair but a matter of degree, a little attention to the subject can pay big dividends. Good nutrition can make us stronger, smarter, and more competent to handle our lives. It can give us power to live.

TABLE OF CONTENTS

CHAPTER 1

WHEN HOPE DIED

"LOOK at yourself. You are disgusting. Your wife will get off the plane from Germany with your baby, look at you, and get back on the plane and go home."

Jerry's* fingers wrapped around the psychologist's ashtray and his knuckles shone white with the ferocity of his grip. He dared not strike back at the inhumanity of the man's comment. This man held a sway over his life that was greater than his own.

Over the last year Jerry had experienced being locked in a padded cell. He had been forced into a straight jacket, and forcibly injected with tranquilizing drugs. He had been taking the most massive amounts of tranquilizing medication the psychiatrists dared to give him for over a year. In addition to this, he had been through a series of shock therapy sessions at a prominent mental hospital. With this therapy an electric current is run through the brain. Afterwards the patient suffers a temporary, but frightening, loss of memory. Because of past experience, Jerry was frightened of the man who sat arrogantly in front of him.

Jerry's mother had walked into the room just prior to the preceeding comments. Tears had run dry over the last year with one sad experience placed solidly on top of another. As she heard the converstation a heavy weight settled about her heart. The previous day she had taken her son out to buy him a new suit to help him feel better about himself. Now the psychiatrist was speaking to him in such a humiliating way. She said to the man, "At least I can be thankful you took him off of drugs."

The psychiatrist said, "I think I'll put him back on his tranquilizing medication Monday." The woman's soul

*Names and circumstances slightly altered to protect the individual involved.

filled with a cold chill. She looked at her son who had gained about 80 pounds as a result of the massive medication he had been on. Everything he did was accomplished in slow motion as a residual effect of the medication he had already been given. The prior psychiatrist had informed the woman that the massive drugs might eventually cause the death of her son if they were continued.

She thought back to how this horrible plight had begun. Her son had worked a year in Berkley with the "down and outers." He had tried to do what he could do to stem the tide of drug abuse and shattered young lives. When he returned he had been suffering from bleeding gums, a sign of malnutrition. After living at home for a while and regaining his strength and health he had traveled to Europe visiting Israel and Germany.

While living in Germany he met Marta, a beautiful young blonde. He proposed on the first date. Eventually she accepted. One day as they were driving on the German road they became involved in an automobile accident. Jerry began to behave in unusual ways after that. His German bride could not understand his behavior. She barely understood his language.

When Jerry's parents were notified of what was going on, they flew him to California. They eagerly awaited him at the San Francisco airport, but he never disembarked. He had wandered off the plane in Los Angeles, thinking the flight was over. For a week he wandered over California.

When Jerry finally entered his parent's home they knew for sure they had a problem. His words made no sense at all. He was taken down for a brain scan which revealed nothing. His behavior was bizarre. Upon one occasion he peeled an orange and banana. He threw the fruit away, blended up the peels in a blender and drank them.

Jerry would sleep late in the dav, but at night he

would come to life. He would often walk or run for miles. One night he was brought home by a couple that lived about 13 miles away from his home. They brought him home because they had compassion for him, even though it was the middle of the night.

Another time Jerry spent the night in a stolen car. The police picked him up and took him to jail. His parents had him released after explaining the situation.

A short time after this Jerry collected all his belongings and went up to the door of a complete stranger. When the couple opened their door, he forced his way in and told them that he was staying with them until he got a job. They were stunned as he dropped his belongings on the floor. They called the police who picked Jerry up and took him to the local psychiatric facility.

When Jerry's parents next saw him he was wrapped in a straight jacket and under great anxiety. All he could think and talk about was his need to get a job to take care of his wife and coming child. Things were now to be taken out of the family's hands. Jerry was to endure a tortured and tragic year of heavy medication and shock therapy. His wife, stranded in Germany, went through the anguish of separation and birth of her child. There would be many long sad days before this loving little family could be reunited again.

As I became involved in these unfolding events I said to myself, "There must be an answer to all this. I am going to look for the answer." I began to look for work at a psychiatric facility and was shortly employed as a psychiatric attendant.

LOCKED UP AND FORGOTTEN

Working at a psychiatric facility can be a very sobering experience. My first realization was that many of these people were not too terribly different from the staff working with them or the people outside of the hospital.

The staff often treated patients with a lack of respect and as things rather than people.

I entered the hospital with a great deal of understanding of the problem and compassion for those suffering from mental illness. Jerry's experience had touched my heart deeply. We had grown up together and I loved him.

The patients at the mental hospital sensed my compassion almost immediately. My shift often began at 11:00 p.m. They would wait up to talk to me. As I walked the halls they would follow me on my rounds, a sight which had an element of humor in it for some. When they learned that I had a relative in a nearby facility they tried to call him and encourage him.

The patients sometimes had their wild moments. I remember turning my back on one fellow. Moments later he picked up a chair and through it through a nearby window.

Staff sometimes treated patients with a lack of understanding. They might become objects of humor or unnecessarily harsh treatment. As a result, several staff were attacked by patients. Sometimes these attacks were seemingly unprovoked.

I began to see patterns. These people who were being locked up together often had a negative impact upon one another. Tempers would flare. One patient would provoke another into a stress reaction.

Self-image emerged as a problem. One young lady had a horrible case of acne. To try to calm her own feelings of worthlessness, she would try to sneak into bed with the male patients. One night we found her slithering along the floor like a snake into the men's quarters.

Many of these people were forgotten. They rarely had visitors. Imagine being incarcerated and forgotten. Most had been in mental hospitals for years, some for most of their lives. People did not know how to handle these people when they did visit. Visitors developed feelings of uneasiness and inability to cope with the situation.

I saw that the plight of these people was hopeless. The hospital had no intentions or ability to improve the lot of these people. They were to be detained, beded and housed. Only by the most unusual of circumstances could one hope to be released. Meanwhile the facility made a healthy profit on each person it housed. Food was the cheapest that could be legally obtained and portions were limited.

The patients were frequently addicted to alcohol, nicotine, coffee and sugar. A regular routine was the hourly intervals at which patients were allowed to smoke a cigarette. They would rush to the counter from every corner of the hospital to "get their smokes."

Bad diet, addiction, stress! The patterns began to sound familiar. I had seen them all with Jerry. He had eaten a poor diet for years. His diet as a youngster contained large amounts of sugar and white flour. The food at the college he attended was typical institutional food. Finally the stress of an automobile accident triggered off a condition of what was being called schizophrenia — it was the straw that broke the camel's back.

After working for eight months at the hospital, I had seen only one patient released. He had purchased some food supplements and started taking them. I quit at this time, realizing that there was not much hope here for helping my friend Jerry.

A thought had been planted in my brain, however. Perhaps part of the explanation for this problem could be traced back to some of the things I had learned in my master's work on fasting.

CHAPTER 2

A FAREWELL TO FAT

I was one of those children who bore a resemblance to Louis XIV of France. In case you do not remember you history lessons, Louis XIV originated the custom of not buttoning the bottom button of his vest. His habit grew out of practicality, not etiquette. Louis made history with his insatiable appetite.

This famous king ate two main meals a day — one at 2:00 p.m. and one at 10:00 at night. A typical meal might begin with 100 oysters for appetizers. This would be followed by 4 large plates of soup.

The next course might by a "Pot-a-Oie." This was a large, fattened goose stuffed with different game birds including pheasants, quail, woodcock, pigeons, ortolans and turtle doves with aromatic herbs. Most people ate only the stuffing, but Louis ate the goose as well.

That was not all of the meal. The King would also eat a whole partridge, a pheasant, plates of vegetables, a selection of salads, two or three thick slices of ham and several helpings of mutton. For dessert he usually ate a plate of assorted cakes and eggs prepared in different ways.

The fork was just coming into vogue at that time, but Louis never adopted it. This was unfortunate for his hat. He lifted his hat when approached by any lady or gentleman while eating. It didn't take long for his hands to become covered with grease, and shortly thereafter his hat became greasy as well.

Toward the end of his regime, Louis developed digestive problems. He eventually lost all of his teeth and spent his last days gumming down moistened bread crumbs.

Autopsy revealed that the king's stomach was 3 times

normal size. Inside the stomach resided an enormous tape worm, living there regally, like some mighty king, and to some extent accounting for the king's enormous appetite.[1]

As a child I was always obese. During my high school and early college years I weighed 210 pounds and had a 38 inch waist. My nickname during my high school years was "The Toad", an appellation which did little for my self-image.

During my third year of college I remember telling my mother that I was always first in line for dinner. Turning to me she said, "From looking at you, I would say you need to be the last in line." Those were cold and harsh words at that time, but I decided to be last in line.

From that time on I quit eating deserts. I began to jog at dinnertime, barely making it for the evening meal. After vigorous exercize my appetite was decreased so I ate less. My weight rapidly dropped to 165 pounds. This happened in 1969 and the weight did not come back. When I first began to jog I could not even travel an eighth of a mile, but soon I was easily able to jog several miles.

One of my areas of interest over the years has been obesity. As has been pointed out, this interest grew out of personal experience. Anyone who has suffered from obesity can't help but have a perpetual interest in the subject. If weight has been lost, keeping it off can be a major concern.

One of my early observations about obesity was the fact that animals in nature are rarely obese. A major effort of the livestock industry has been to fatten animals for the marketplace. I wondered if perhaps an understanding of how animals are fattened would be helpful in understanding human obesity.

CATTLE FATTENED FOR SLAUGHTER

This writer has never seen a treatise comparing the technology which has been developed for fattening domestic animals for slaughter with the tremendous human problem of obesity which we face. In reality, there are several parallels. What we have intensionally done to our cattle (and other domestic animals) we have unintensionally and ignorantly done to ourselves in many instances. We have fattened ourselves for the slaughter of heart disease and other executioners.

One of the techniques used to fatten cattle is to stuff them with concentrated carbohydrate foods. Such animals are called "grain fed" and have more fat than grass fed animals. People frequently fatten themselves with concentrated carbohydrate and fatty foods. All of the following foods are rich in calories and tend to promote weight gain: sugar, white flour, fried foods, milk, butter and margarine, crackers, roasted and salted nuts. This is only a brief sampling of many of our favorite foods. No wonder many of us have become as obese as our cattle! Did you ever try to gain weight on a diet of celery, string beans and lettuce? It is impossible.

Livestock raisers have also discovered that the hormone balance of their animals can be intensionally upset in such a way as to promote weight gain and marbling of fat through the body. DES, a synthetic female hormone, has been used for this purpose even though it is a potential carcinogen (cancer causing substance) and residues of the hormone have been found in the livers of implanted animals.[2] Millions of Americans have upset hormone balances due to taking birth control pills, postmenopausal estrogens, eating large amounts of sugar, or lack of certain nutrients including the essential fatty acids and zinc.

A final secret in fattening livestock is not to allow them to exercize. It is very difficult to promote weight gain on animals that are exercising. Lack of exercise, however, changes the whole chemistry of the body, promoting weight gain. Most Americans lead very sedentary lives. We have forgotten the art of walking.

NUTRITION AND OBESITY

It is the usual practice of many people in their attempts to lose weight to forget about one of the most important factors involved at the very outset. Unfortunately and to my own detriment, it is something I was completely unaware of in my own weight loss program. The body is a very delicately balanced organism, designed to operate on a very special kind of fuel. The materials which a person consumes in his diet furnish the building blocks which the body has available for the building up of itself.

A person may undergo all manner of external attempts to develop a lithe, well-muscled body, but if nutrition is inadequate such efforts will be of no avail. Exercise is very important in coping with obesity, as will be discussed later, but without concern about nutrition it can be downright dangerous.

Exercize is a catabolic (tearing down) process. The ability of the body to build itself up after exercise (anabolism) will be directly linked to quality of the diet which is consumed. The ability of the body to rebuild and renew itself after exercise would not be greatly facilitated by a diet of soda pop and french fries.

Many Americans stuff themselves with foods which are high in calories, but low in real quality, simply because they are the foods which are the most readily available. There is no difficulty walking into a convenient shop and obtaining bread, ice cream, coffee, starchy foods of every description, sugary foods, and pre-packaged meals. These are the foods one needs to watch carefully to lose weight. It is not as easy or as popular to dine upon yeast, whole grains, sprouts, raw nuts, fish, and fresh fruits and vegetables.

The simple dietary change outlined above was the first step I took in my own personal attempt to lose weight. I am of the opinion that this simple change would help a great many other people.

Every individual has an inborn appetite control mechanism. If this were not so a person would eat himself to death with his first meal. It stands to reason that if this mechanism is seriously undernourished it could easily cause a person to continue eating beyond what he should in the hopes of obtaining the nutriment his body needs. Thus there is possibly a certain extent to which quantity will be overlooked by the appetite control mechanism of the brain in the search for quality. This can mean a weight gain. It is hopeless to try to lose weight without a healthy and well-nourished appetite control mechanism on one's side.

The all important role that proper nutrition could play in weight control has been summarized by Dr. Roger Williams:

> We know that optimal nutrition as a means of permanently controlling weight gain would, if approached properly, put every fad diet in the discard heap, where they collectively belong. For adults, the trouble with fad diets is that without exception they fail to consider the tremendous variations in *individual* requirements, and instead mistakenly identify certain foods as good for *all* people. When will responsible research programs put a stop to the try-a-new-weight-loss-diet-each-week mania that has for so long — and so futilely — afflicted us? Doctors have never properly investigated what supernutrition could do to keep healthy our appestat (the glandular mechanism that controls the body's desire for food) and the brain's "activity center" (another such mechanism

that impels us to take needed exercise): properly nourished, the appestat and activity center could work together to prevent obesity or institute long lasting weight control. (Dr. Roger Williams, "Fighting for Real Nutrition".)

BIOCHEMICAL IMBALANCE

As has been pointed out, cattle are often fattened by giving them female hormones. The purpose of a DES implant is to fill the muscle of the animal with fat, so that it will be tender and juicy. The biochemical imbalances that human beings suffer can produce obesity in much the same way.

The first hormone imbalance which millions of American women have subjected themselves to is the intake of estrogens similar to those implanted in cattle. The following is a comment made on oral contraceptives in a manual on prescription drugs:

> Possible Side-Effects (natural, expected, and unavoidable drug actions). Retention of fluid, *gain in weight*[3] . . . (Emphasis added).

The very same comment is made under the heading of estrogens, which are not only widely used to prevent contraception, but for other purposes as well.

An individual does not have to ingest estrogen in order to have high estrogen levels in his body. The following is a summary of urine hormone residue studies of young American athletes on the "usual training-table diet":

> THE ESTROGENS:
>
> 10.0 mcgm. normal. In every case, the first or initial study showed approximately two times this quantity . . .
>
> *Significance:* High estrogen values in the male show a trend toward the slowing down of muscle formation and a stepping up of fat deposition.

This aberration is part of the reason for the tendency of middle-aged men to replace muscle with fat. That a trend in this direction should be uncovered by biochemical tests of young athletes is disturbing.[4]

The implication of this study is that the "average American diet" with its overly processed foods may very well be contributing to hormone imbalance and thus to obesity. The estrogen levels of these athletes were lowered to normal by supplementing their diets with grain concentrates.

A second biochemical imbalance which can directly affect one's ability to maintain a reasonable weight or to lose weight is blood insulin levels. Ordinarily, insulin levels fluctuate very little in the body. When insulin levels fluctuate wildly they can contribute to a weight problem.

Simple sugars are the primary culprits in creating insulin imbalances, but caffein and alcohol can also play an important role. It has been discovered that refined carbohydrates produce two to five times more blood fat than do unrefined carbohydrates. This may very well be a result of the fact that simple sugars cause significantly higher levels of insulin in the blood.[5]

High levels of fat in the blood tend to promote obesity as well as other health problems. One of the objectives of a sensible weight loss program should be to *decrease blood fat* and *blood insulin* levels, which are high due to sugar in the diet. Once these are lowered a pathway is opened for the body to burn stored fat in the muscles.

A final imbalance which should be remedied for weight loss is the absence of fiber in the diet. If the diet is high in fiber the body can dump excess fats from the body in the form of bile acids. Bile acids are fatty digestive substances whose secretion is increased by a high fiber diet. There is also evidence that a high roughage diet impairs the ability of the intestine to absorb calories.[6] Fiber content of the diet should ideally come from whole foods.

EXERCISE AND OBESITY

DANGERS OF EXERCISE

Lafayette Jogger Dies
Lesher News Bureau

Lafayette — A Lafayette woman jogging at the Lafayette reservoir Saturday afternoon collapsed and died before her parents and son, coroner's deputies said.[7]

The above story is not new to the history of jogging. One of the first recorded jogs took place in 490 B.C. when a young Greek soldier named Pheidippides ran from the plains of Marathon to the city of Athens — a distance of some 26 miles — with the news that the Persian army had been defeated in their attempt to conquor the Greek world. Unfortunately, after shouting, "Rejoice, we conquer!" he fell over dead ![8]

Those who enter upon a hastily considered exercize program can run a tremendous risk as illustrated above. The question which arises is why such a natural activity should be fraught with any danger at all. One puzzles because the famous Framingham study concluded in 1971 showed that the death rate from heart disease was five times less among physically active men than among inactive men.[9]

The dangers of exercise are a result of the fact that many Americans suffer from blockage of the coronary arteries. When these arteries which supply the heart with oxygen become clogged a dangerous situation can develop.

A heart with a good blood supply has a healthy pink

color. When a coronary artery becomes clogged, the part of the heart affected will become starved for oxygen and develop a bluish color. A person with atherosclerosis might have one part of the heart a healthy pink and another part an oxygen starved blue.

Where a blue area and a pink area meet an *oxygen differential line* forms. This indicates a major difference in the amount of oxygen reaching the two sides of the line.

An evenly oxygenated heart is not very likely to fail, even if it is poorly oxygenated. The heart muscle may die, however, if it is all blue for too long.

The problem arises when a heart is checker-boarded with areas of blue and pink. This pattern may develop when a person is at rest. It is much more likely, however, that it will develop as a result of exercise. Strenuous exertion can so increase the demand of the heart for oxygen that blue and pink oxygen differentials show, due to partial blockage of some of the coronary arteries.

It has been found that the heart muscle contracts better on the high side of an oxygen differential line than on the low side. This can cause the heart muscle to be thrown into a spasm of fluttering or uncoordinated trembling in place of a strong coordinated rhythm. This is the very common type of heart attack called a fibrillation.[10]

This risk can be greatly reduced by introducing exercise slowly and building it up gradually. Exercise will increase oxygenation of the heart by both increasing the size of coronary arteries and also allowing new arteries to grow to replace those that have been blocked. Thus exercise can become a life saving rather than life concluding event.[11]

One of the keys to avoiding excesses in exercise is called "pulse-monitored exercise." The heart has a maximum rate at which it can beat which varies with age. A person with a possible problem of atherosclerosis and coronary artery blockage (which includes most of us) should not exercise at more than 75 percent of this maximum capacity. Those without this problem can exercise the heart at 80 percent of capacity, while a trained athlete can safely work the heart at 85 percent of capacity.[12]

The jogging pace necessary to produce a 75 percent of maximum pulse rate is not strenuous, but rather a moderate, comfortable, and easy to achieve level of exercise.[13] It is possible to be in such poor shape that merely lifting the heels off the ground is exercise sufficient to produce a 75 percent of maximum pulse rate.[14]

People over 40 or those with a heart problem should have a stress electrocardiogram before starting and exercise program. This is a test of the ability of the heart to function during exercise. It can reliably indicate the risk of a heart attack during exercise.[15]

THE TRAINING EFFECT

The goal of exercise for the best overall physical fitness should be what is called the "training effect." The "training effect" is a result of aerobic exercise, that is an exercise in which the body uses large amounts of oxygen for an extended period of time.

When speaking of the "training effect" one is concerned with the changes in the body which occur as a result of exercise. There are changes in respiration, in the heart and circulatory system, and in the muscles.

Aerobic exercise strengthens the muscles of respiration. This makes it easier for air to flow into and out of the lungs. Poor respiration can cripple the rest of the body.

The strength of the heart is also increased by aerobic exercise. The heart gains the ability to pump more blood with each stroke. This means that oxygen can be carried more easily to all the cells of the body. Transportation of nutrients is also improved.

Aerobic exercise increases the total amount of blood circulating through the body. The number of red blood cells and amount of oxygen carrying hemoglobin increases.[16] New capillary arteries and other routes of blood flow are opened up, which can cause a drop in high blood pressure.[17]

Muscles are toned by aerobic exercise. There is usually an increase in percentage of the body that is muscle and a decrease in the percentage of the body that is fat. A person who is engaging in aerobic exercise has muscles that not only burn more calories when exercising, but also burn more calories when he is inactive than does a non-exerciser.[18]

DETERMINATION OF YOUR EXERCISE LEVEL

A person's maximum pulse rate varies according to age. A 20 year-old will have a pulse rate of 210 but the rate slows down about one beat per minute per year thereafter. This is based on an average pulse of 72 for males and 80 for females. To obtain a training effect a person needs to engage in aerobic exercise which will raise the pulse to between 75 and 80 percent of maximum for about 20 minutes.

A person with a history of heart disease or a potential problem in this area should aim for the lower level of exercise. If the pulse is more than 12 beats per minute below average the exercise formula given below will have to be altered (See Footnote)[19]

COMPUTING IDEAL PULSE FOR AEROBIC EXERCISE:

Maximum Heartbeat	210
Minus Years Over 20	10
Maximum Pulse for My Age	200

200 x 75% = 150 beats per minute

SOME SAMPLE COMPUTATIONS:

Age	Maximum Pulse	75% Minimum Pulse Rate	80% Maximum Pulse Rate
20	210	158	168
25	205	154	164
30	200	150	160
35	195	147	156
40	190	143	152
45	185	139	148
50	170	128	136
55	165	124	132
60	160	120	128
65	155	117	124

EXERCISE AND FAT

Fat accumulates not only in rolls around the middle, but also can replace muscle which atrophies as a result of disuse. This latter is called intramuscular fat. The person who has a large roll around the middle will also have large quantities of intramuscular fat.

A person's ability to exercise aerobically will be dependent to a large extent upon how much of his body is fat. Ideally, men should not have more than 15 percent of the body as fat, and women should not have more than 22 percent fat. It is not uncommon for men to average 23 percent fat and women 36 percent fat.[20]

The percentage of fat on the body can be determined by weighing the body under water. Fat floats, so the less a person weighs under water the more fat he has in his body and the less muscle and bone. A very rough guess of your percentage of fat can be made as follows:

More than 25% fat — A person will float easily; 22-23% fat — A person will float while breathing shallowly ; 15% fat — A person will sink slowly with a full chest of air; 13% fat or less — A person will sink readily, even with a full chest of air, even in salt water.[21]

Muscle is the major fat burning portion of the body. The brain does this only under the unusual circumstance of fasting. Therefore, building the muscle mass of the body through exercise makes it easier for the body to burn fat. This means that regular aerobic exercise should be a major component of any weight reduction or maintenance program. Even more important, it is the best way to say farewell to unwanted fat.

The duration of aerobic exercise is important for obtaining maximum benefits. A few years ago a team of doctors studied several groups of young men who ran for different periods of time on a treadmill. Times varied from 10 minutes to 40 minutes. The researchers found measurable improvement in cardiovascular fitness in those who ran for 20 minutes or longer, while there was little improvement in those who ran less than 20 minutes.[22] Some maintain that a training effect can be obtained with only 12 minutes of exercise a day, but it would be a tragedy to lose the full benefit of one's exercise because duration of the exercise was inadequate.

Lack of exercise is known to promote obesity. When rats, which do not normally become obese, are put in a warm, small cage they invariably become obese. They can eventually come to weigh two or three times as much as rats allowed to exercise. Animals kept in cool cages do not have as much tendency to gain weight.

(The winter energy crisis may save us yet if we keep our thermostats down.) These rat experiments simply substantiate the long recognized practical experience of farmers. When they want to fatten geese, cattle, or hogs for butchering they are commonly confined and not allowed to exercise.[23]

SOME OTHER CONSIDERATIONS

FREQUENT CONSUMPTION OF SMALL AMOUNTS OF FOOD

Prolonged abstinence from food tends to produce gorging. This could be both a biological and psychological problem. Rats have been shown to become obese if they were allowed to eat only one meal a day, weighing 30 percent more after three weeks than rats allowed to nibble to satisfy their hunger.[24] One's body feels less need to store reserves of fat if it is biologically convinced that food is not very far away or very hard to get.

EMOTIONAL FACTORS IN OVEREATING

Emotions can contribute to a problem of weight control in several ways. Emotions can alter hormone levels in the body. Feelings of inhibition and insecurity or boredom or excessive pressure can cause a person to try to eat out his or her frustrations. Unfortunately, eating does not solve emotional problems, but it can intensify them.

Internal motivations for overating can be very difficult to deal with. The desire to lose weight must come from within a person, it is impossible to impose it from without.

BLAND DIET

A rich and exotic diet produces a far greater tendency

to overeat than does a bland one. A simple, adequate, and bland diet is best for weight loss. Self-restraint can easily disappear if refined foods laced with sugar and spices are included in the diet.

ALLERGIES AND OBESITY

Two kinds of allergies can contribute to obesity. The brain contains an appetite control center in the area known as the hypothalmus. In this area are "turn-on-appetite" cells and "turn-off-appetite" cells. Both of these can be influenced by stimulants, depressants, and allergies.

Many people are aware of how an allergy can swell the sinuses shut and make it difficult to breathe. It is possible for a chemical or an allergen to alter the functioning of the "turn-off-appetite" cells in the brain. Two scientists from the National Institute of Health found that by injections of a common experimental chemical they could cause laboratory mice to overeat and grow fat. Autopsy revealed permanent damage to the "turn-off-appetite" cells.[25]

Some drugs such as tranquilizers affect the "turn-off-appetite" cells and cause people on them to overeat and become obese. Nutritional deficiencies can work in a similar way. We know that protein deficiency of a mother during the first three months of pregnancy will damage the appetite control mechanism of the child's brain and result in an obese child.[26]

A person whose "turn-off-appetite" cells have been damaged by a food or chemical he eats may well go on an eating rampage. He may be unable to stop eating until he has eaten everyting in sight.

An allergist is often able to reproduce this hunger by

placing the substance that triggers the hunger under the tongue. This is called sublingual allergy testing.

A second form of "allergy" which can promote obesity is one which stimulates the "turn-on-appetite" cells. Some substances when placed in the body create a desire for themselves. Sometimes there will be a withdrawal if the substance is not obtained on a regular basis as is the case with heroine addiction. It is possible to have a heroin-like addiction to certain foods like sugar.

In other situations the stimulation of the "turn-on-appetite" cells is not as enslaving. Simple sight and smell of food can stimulate these cells. The taste of sweetness and spices can stimulate appetite. I am writing these words the day after Thanksgiving, full well realizing that the spices and sugar in the dressing and pumpkin pie stimulated my "turn-on-appetite" cells, causing me to eat far more food than is rational or sensible.

It is almost a universal human experience for sugar and spices to stimulate appetite and cause overeating. Less frequently, a person's appetite may be overstimulated by wheat or yeast or some other food substance. Avoiding these substances can result in pronounced weight loss.

SUPPLEMENTATION FOR WEIGHT LOSS

This section is written with the assumption that a person will wish to include aerobic exercise as a part of his or her weight loss program. Exercise is a catabolic activity. This means that it "tears down" the body. For this reason supplementation should be of such a nature that it both enables the body to rebuild itself and also maximizes the ability of a person to carry on physical activity.

Supplements valuable from these standpoints are as

follows:

1. A Lipotropic Adjunct — (lipo - fat, tropic - to eat, adjunct - helper). A combination of nutrients such as choline, inositol, lipase, betaine, methionine, and B12 will help the body use dietary and cellular fats. These nutrients convert blood and cellular fats into a more water soluble form enabling them to be better burned, used, or excreted by the body.

During exercise the body burns a lot of fat in the muscle. This supplement can facilitate the process. Dr. William Hose has stated that a good lipotropic adjunct can be as much as thirty times more effective than lecithin which works in the body in a similar way.[27]

2. Vitamin E — Vitamin E, like the lipotropic adjunct, decreases the risk of a heart attack while exercising. It is a vasodialator opening the smaller arteries so that more blood and oxygen can flow through them. This oxygenation of the body reduces the risk of oxygen differential lines and a heart attack.

Vitamin E also increases the strength and endurance of muscle tissue. A frog heart removed from the animal will beat 50 percent longer if placed in a vitamin E solution than if placed in a saline solution. Vitamin E treated rats can swim twice as long as animals not given E. They can withstand high altitiudes which kill untreated animals. Human beings tested on a treadmill also show increased endurance with vitamin E supplementation[28]

3. Octacosanol — This is a rather exotic substance found in wheat germ, sardines and California herring. It is a waxy alcohol readily destroyed by heat (as in toasting wheat germ).

Twenty years of controlled studies with over a thousand people have shown that this substance benefits exercisers. It improves stamina and endurance, reduces heart stress and quickens reaction time.[29] Octacosanol would be a natural component of a wheat germ concentrate.

4. Dessicated Liver — Dr. B.H. Ershoff conducted some remarkable experiments with this substance and found that liver does indeed contain "anti-fatigue" factors. Dr. Ershoff divided 60 rats into 3 groups. For 12 weeks one group received all they wanted of a basic "balanced" diet. A second group received the same "balanced diet" fortified with vitamins, while a third group received the same diet as group two with the addition of 10 percent dried liver.

After 12 weeks the rats were tested for endurance by dropping them, one by one, in a tank of water from which they could not escape. Swimming thus became the test for strength and endurance. Rats in the first group swam an average of 13.3 minutes before drowning. Group 2 did little better. In the third group one rat swam 60 minutes, another 83 minutes and another 87 minutes. The nine other rats in the group were able to swim almost 10 times as long as the rats in the other two groups. The study indicates the contribution liver can make to exercisers who seek to improve energy and endurance.[30] If we can exercise longer we can burn fat off the body more readily.

The liver of an animal detoxifies poisons of the body. Liver which is consumed should not come from an animal which has been exposed to herbicides, pesticides and synthetic female hormones like DES. DES implants in the ears of cattle can result in liver residues of the substance.[31] Some companies obtain their liver supplements from other countries where cattle are not exposed to these toxic substances.

Rancidity is a real problem with a liver supplement. This can cause a strong taste and smell. To prevent this liver supplements are sometimes defatted, saturated with vitamin C and/or encapsulated in a protein shell to prevent contact of fats and other substances with oxygen.

REBOUND EXERCISE

A majority of joggers have a medical history of physical damage related to jogging. This is usually due to what is known as "the jarring effect" of exercising on a hard surface. In nature hard surfaces are rare. Anywhere that plants will grow (which would be the only places man could survive), the soil would be intermixed with rich deposits of decaying organic matter. Rich light topsoil would extend into the earth for 9 - 18 inches or more. This is the kind of surface the human foot was designed to exercise on.

A relatively new form of exercise known as rebound exercise is designed to duplicate the pattern we find in nature. Rebound exercise is accomplished by bouncing up and down on a surface which has some give to it. The trampoline developed in 1939 was the first commercially available instrument for rebound exercise. More recently instruments similar to miniature trampolines have been marketed.

Rebound exercise can provide the benefits of jogging without the physical damage which can result when a person jogs on pavement or some other hard surface. It seems that the human body was designed for this. Rebounding is a relatively safe and efficient way to exercise.

CHAPTER 3

FASTING: LEARNING NOT TO EAT

AS a result of my experience with obesity in childhood and young adulthood I developed a continuing interest not only in eating and obesity but also in the whole idea of refraining from food or fasting. I lost my weight in my third year of college. A couple of years later while at Dallas Theological Seminary I first heard about fasting. I was fascinated . . .

My faculty advisor looked at me in a rather peculiar way. I had just informed him that I wished to do my master's work in the area of fasting. Such an idea was quite foreign to him at that time. Seminary students ordinarily invested their time in the pursuit of answers to theological questions. He rather cautiously gave his approval to the study.

It did not take me long to realize that physical discipline was an integral part of the lives of the early Christians. Christ had fasted for 40 days prior to his ministry. Paul was no stranger to fasting. I still found myself wondering what happened in the body when a person quit eating.

Around this time I learned of a prominent fasting clinic in central Texas. This clinic had guided thousands of people through long fasts. I arranged to visit with the head of the clinic and to talk with some of the patients who had undertaken long fasts. This was the beginning of an interest and investigation of one of the most beneficial practices that a person can undertake. Eventually fasting would help me to better understand schizophrenia and similiar problems.

FORTY-THREE DAYS WITHOUT FOOD

It was a warm July afternoon. We sat a short distance from a two story cream colored building situated on the top of a hill. A large balcony on the second floor of the building looked out upon the chairs and benches where we sat.

I sat near a middle aged woman and a young Jewish girl. I was speaking to the middle aged woman, "Mrs. S. how long did you fast?"

"I fasted a total of forty-three days," she replied. "During this time I lost thirty-four pounds."

"What were some of your experiences during your fast?" I asked.

"I lost my voice on the second day of the fast and did not regain it for fifty-seven days. As a matter of fact I regained my voice this morning."

"My interview with you is rather well timed then," I commented.

"Yes, indeed," she said. I noted the slow deliberateness with which she spoke. She seemed very relaxed and rested. "I had other experiences as well during my fast. I had very bad headaches which I think were due to a withdrawal from my addiction to coffee. Prior to fasting I had been a heavy coffee drinker."

I was surprised that a person would go through withdrawal reactions from such a commonly used and seemingly harmless substance as coffee. Many years later a medical doctor would share an article from the Journal of the American Medical Association describing how withdrawal from coffee often results in headaches for several days. My mind would wander back to this incident.

"My tongue was coated with thick white paste," she continued, and I had to shower twice a day in order to remove a strong odor on my skin. During the last seven days of my fast I developed the dry heaves. After breaking my fast I had a period of numbness in my mouth and arms for about half an hour, but the head of the institution assured me it would go away and it did."

"What did you think about while you were fasting?", I inquired.

"I thought about food all the time, even though I was not hungry. I did a lot of reading in order to get my mind off food."

"Why did you decide to go on such a long fast?" I queried.

"My husband is a Greek Orthodox Priest. He once fasted for seven days. There is much fasting in the Greek Orthodox seminaries, or at least there was until fairly recently. This was the source of my information and interest in fasting. I came here hoping to have my goiter go away. As you can see it is still there."

For the first time I noticed the large benign growth on her neck. Her conversation had been so engaging that it had completely blinded me to the obvious physical deformity she suffered from.

"I was told not to expect the goiter to go away with one long fast, but I understand that there is a good chance it will go away with several additional shorter fasts."

"I hope it does," I said, although the whole notion was quite foreign to me.

"Did you have any vivid dreams while fasting?" I asked this question because my academic study had shown that fasting had been part of the puberty rites of some primitive peoples. They would send their young men out into the forest to fast until they had a dream or a vision, whereupon they would be accepted into the tribe. I wondered if perhaps the functioning of the brain was not altered to make dreams more vivid as it burned fat during the process of fasting.

"My dreams are always vivid," she said. "I did have a prophetic dream of when I would eat again. My husband had visions when he fasted."

"How did you break your fast?"

"I broke my fast with two ounces of orange juice every two hours. The orange juice was too sweet so I switched to grapefruit juice."

Since this time it has been learned that it is better to break a fast with whole foods in most instances, since the fiber restores the operation of the digestive tract more rapidly.

THIRTY NINE DAYS WITHOUT FOOD

While this conversation had been taking place the beautiful young Jewish girl lounging in the sun nearby indicated an obvious interest in sharing her story.

"Would you like to tell me about your fast?", I asked.

"Oh, yes" she replied. "I fasted for 39 days. I had plenty of energy during my fast and was not hungry, although I thought a lot about food. After four weeks I became uncomfortable and nauseous. I began to develop sinus problems. After thirty-nine days I became exhausted and nervous."

"Why did you come here?" I inquired.

"I came here as a heavy smoker with a lymphatic disorder called lymphodema. My leg had been swollen for over six months. There is an operation for the condition, but it has not been very successful and I didn't really want to try it."

"I was quite disappointed that the swelling did not go away during the fast."

Looking at her sun tanned legs I could see no indication whatsoever of swelling. She continued, "Fortunately, after I resumed eating the healthy diet provided here the condition disappeared."

I remembered looking at her in amazement. Earlier that day the head of the clinic had told me they flew their food in fresh from Hawaii. Food was eaten raw with the exception of two steamed vegetables a day. This was my first faint realization of the fact that what a person eats is as important as what he does not eat. I had long before realized the value of exclusion of sugar and other harmful substances from the diet, but the idea of including foods in the diet that would help the body to function better first began to form at this moment.

The young lady continued, "I had a great deal of difficulty in stopping smoking, but it was not allowed on the fast. I spit up mucus during my fast. This was probably due to the accumulated residues of my smoking. At any rate, the fast made my sense of taste, smell and hearing much keener."

"Thank you for your story," I said.

One point stood out in my memory as I thought back on my experiences with fasting as it applied to my relative's suffering. The Russians had been able to help 70% of those suffering from mental illness by removing them from food. I asked myself the meaning of this, but the significance was not yet clear.

THE BEAR AND THE BUTTERFLY

The story is told of a restaurant manager who addressed a waiter in a slightly irritated manner and said, "George, why did that man from the table over in the corner get up and leave so suddenly?"

The waiter replied, "Well sir, he sat down and asked for hot dogs. I told him that we were out of them, but that if he would wait a few minutes I would get the cook to make some."

"What happened then?" asked the manager.

The waiter resumed his story, "I went to the kitchen and accidentally stepped on the dog's tail. It yelped out. The man got up and left."

Fasting is an unusual occurrence to the western mind. Many people have imbued it with strange and mystical significance. Actually, as the above illustration clearly demonstrates, often times people have very simple and easily explainable reasons for going without food.

We are frequently led by others to think that fasting is a rare and uncommon occurrence. This is not really the case. Fasting is always going on in nature. The bear is a good example. During the abundant summer months he stores away a good supply of fat to keep him alive during the lean, snow drenched winter months. The hibernation of the bear and other animals is really nothing more or less than the practice of fasting in nature.

Everyone is familiar with the hump of the camel, which many think holds water. Actually, the hump is a reserve food supply as well. If a camel is put on slim rations the hump will fall flat on the back.

Another example of an animal with a specialized part of the body for storing food is the fat-tailed sheep of Persia. During times of plenty the sheep stores up large quantities of food in its tail. Prize specimens can develop such heavy tails that the owners place small carts under the tails to prevent them from dragging on the ground. When pasturage becomes scarce the sheep draw upon the reserves in their tails.[2]

The male Alaskan fur seal does not eat or sleep during June, July and August. This is his mating season. At the end of this time he is a physical wreck as one might well imagine. He will then wiggle into the tall grass away from the beach and sleep for three weeks. Only then does he wake up and begin to worry about food.[3]

You may never have seen an Alaskan fur seal, a camel or even a bear. Even so, you have probably still run into a fasting organism. Many plants go into a dormancy period during the winter and are then renewed in the spring. The potato and the onion, with tuber and bulb, are good examples.

Take a cutting from a fig tree or a grape vine some

time. It need have no leaves or roots, yet without these it has no way of receiving nourishment. Given water these cuttings will produce leaves and roots. In other words a transfer of material can take place within the cutting, there is both a tearing down and also a building up.

A caterpillar forms a cacoon and entering it goes into a fast. Enzymes completely break down the tissues of the caterpillar, as anyone would know who has opened up a cacoon. Yet the tissues are reassembled to form a butterfly. This has to be one of the most amazing phenomena in nature.

The purpose of this little introduction to fasting is twofold. Firstly, it is to demonstrate that fasting is not a rare and uncommon occurrence. Secondly, it is to show that fasting is not purely destructive, that it can be a constructive and renewing process.

WHY DO PEOPLE FAST?

There are at least three basic reasons why people fast.

The first reason why people have fasted historically is political. Gandhi fasted in order to persuade the British to grant independence to India. One of the interesting sidelights here is that fasting for political reasons has been used most frequently against the British and the Americans. The reason for this is that these peoples are generally unfamiliar with the idea of fasting. To go without food is an unthinkable ordeal for the average American. This makes him very vulnerable to those who would use fasting as a tool for political ends.

A second reason why people have fasted is for religious reasons. Fasting was a frequent occurance in the Bible.

The Zulus have no faith in a fat prophet.[4] In religious literature fasting is frequently involved with dreams or visions. It has been frequently practiced in order to influence the supernatural world.

A third reason why people fast is to promote good health. In fasting literature the practice has been noted to be frequently beneficial for respiratory and digestive problems. These are two key avenues of nutrition for the body. We obtain oxygen through the lungs, and nutrients through the digestive tract. It is not surprising, then, that if these two functions are helped people experience a general improvement in health.

WHEN HUNGER DIES

Dr. Buchinger likens fasting to the situation of an Alaskan farmer cut off by winter snowdrifts. As fuel supplies run low the farmer is forced to use progressively more valuable combustible material to keep himself warm. He will begin by burning spare lumber, old magazines and trash, but in the end he will be forced to put the ax to his fine mahogany furniture and place it into the fire in order to keep himself warm.

This analogy is applied to fasting in the following way:

> The more inferior the material the less compunction there is about burning it in the fire of metabolism. Gradually, however, after deposits of fat, impurities and degenerated tissue have been consumed, the body substance can no longer be treated so generously . . . The delicate inner mechanism carries out work of amazing detail, like a surgeon operating without a knife. In this phase dangerous and stubborn deposits are mostly attacked. Only if the hidden corners have been cleaned out, does the organism have to approach valuable remaining areas of flesh to maintain its metabolism while fasting.[5]

In a very rough and general way it is possible to divide a fast into several stages. These are as follows:

Stage One:

One to three days in which the body is living off of immediate reserves. Hunger is present.

Stage Two:

A change to "ketosis" or "fat metabolism". Normally the body nourishes the brain and nervous system and muscles with glucose or sugar. During fasting the body has the ability to change body chemistry. The body begins to nourish the brain and nervous system with particles of fat called "ketones". Anyone who has eaten a lot of fat knows that it supresses hunger. Hunger ceases during this stage of fasting. The change will take place from two to six days after fasting begins. Physical hunger is as supressed as if you were to eat a cube of butter. Psychological hunger will still be present.

Stage Three:

A feeling of increasing well being. This is only for healthy individuals. A person who is not well can experience some truly frightening symptoms during this phase of fasting. Because of the many toxic substances in the environment and food supply most twentieth century Americans find it difficult to conduct a normal fast.

Stage Four:

The return of hunger occurs. This happens at the point when the fat of the body has been burned for energy. This hunger is a keen sharp hunger which will not go away and is manifest in the nose, mouth and throat rather than in the stomach. A very fat person may have no return of hunger within a reasonable period of time because of all the fat which can be burned on the body. Ordinarily hunger will return within 30 to 60 days.

Stage Five:

Starvation and death take place if the fast is not broken soon after hunger returns. The body begins to tear apart precious tissues composed of protein in order to go on living.

That hunger dies during a fast has been well known since ancient times. We are told in the pages of the New Testament that Jesus Christ fasted forty days and forty nights and afterwards he was hungry.

SYMPTOMS DURING FASTING

Fasting is frequently associated with various physical symptoms. Abdominal discomfort and emptiness can result in sleeplessness. Nausea and dry heaves can occur, particularly if a person is quite toxic. Headache and dizziness are common. A person will frequently feel dizzy and weak when standing rapidly. The tongue becomes coated white during the early part of a fast. As the fast continues the tongue will frequently become clear and pink.

The body can also become quite sensitive to cold while going without food. When I lived in Dallas I would frequently fast during the long hot summer days. At these times the heat did not bother me, while at other times it was quite unbearable.

Some of the symptoms experienced during fasting are beneficial and pleasant. Weight loss is an obvious accompaniment of fasting. A person will frequently note improvement of the senses of smell, hearing and taste. Respiration can improve dramatically during fasting. Fasting also provides an opportunity for withdrawal from allergens and addictions. Many physicians are now using fasting to detect food allergy problems. Patients are put on a short fast with distilled water for several days. Foods are then gradually introduced. If a patient is allergic to a food reactions are very swift and dramatic.

THE RISKS OF FASTING

There are risks associated with fasting for the very simple reason that toxic substances are being dumped from the body during the fast. Paul Bragg tells the story of how on one occassion he undertook a twenty-one day fast. "On the 19th day I had terrible pains in my bladder — when I urinated it felt like red hot water passing through me. I had the urine examined and sure enough it was filled with DDT and other deadly pesticide poisons.[6]

DDT is stored in the fat of the body as are some other potentially harmful and deadly substances. When they are released into the system during fasting they can have very unpleasant side effects. They will be released as fat is used to nourish the body during the fast. DDT has been found to contaminate even the bodies of those people who live in the most remote corners of the globe.

Linda Clark has summarized this problem rather pointedly as follows:

> As the fatty tissues, where the insecticides are stored, begin to break down, the poisons are released into the blood stream. They become your sole "nourishment." Thus you can poison yourself. For this reason, total fasting has caused illness, occasional death.
>
> Yet insecticides are only one of the many poisons we are exposed to daily. Other poisons are stored in the body, too. When you fast you are providing your body with an undiluted menu of poisons.[7]

There are other toxic substances stored in the body in addition to pesticides. For example, metabolic wastes can accumulate within cells. Cells are not destroyed during fasting, rather they shrink in size. Waste products stored in the cells are eliminated during this process.

It is probable that minerals are withdrawn from the bones during a prolonged fast. There are also dangerous substances such as lead, strontium and fluoride which can accumulate in bones.

It is because of these risks that many recommend only short fasts or juice fasting. It is for these reasons that adequate quantities of liquids should be consumed during fasting, so that the body can wash out toxins and waste products. A longer fast will increase the risks of fasting and should be supervised by someone competent in the area.

FASTING AND AGING

Dr. Alexis Carrel, author of *Man, The Unknown*, kept fragments of a chicken heart alive for years. He learned that if cells were not kept free of their own cell waste they aged rapidly. If cell wastes were regularly washed away the cells did not age. As cell wastes are washed out of the body during fasting, the cells are enabled to stay younger longer.[8]

One of the characteristics of aging is a slowdown in the metabolic rate. Everything that happens in the body takes place more slowly than it would in a younger person. I frequently think of this when I am driving on the freeway. Many older persons drive very slowly. I, at the present time being a little bit younger, wish to travel a little bit faster.

Anything which will increase the metabolic rate making all reactions taking place in the body occur a little bit more rapidly will actually reverse aging. A fast of thirty to forty days will increase the rate of body metabolism by 5-6 per cent. Exercise and nutrition also have the capability for increasing metabolic rate.[9]

Fasting is, in a sense, the fountain of youth for which men have sought from time immemorial. Many of the longest living persons in the world have either fasted often, or consumed very small quantities of food. A man named Tara Singh of India underwent a forty-eight day fast for political reasons in 1960. Physicians observing him felt that the seventy-six year old man had increased his life span by at least ten years as a result of the fast.[10]

One of the interesting observations which has been made with regard to aging is that mammals normally live about six times their maturation period. A dog that matures in two years will usually live twelve years. Man on the other hand averages only three times his maturation period. He matures in about 20 years and usually lives to about 60. Improved diet and fasting might improve this record considerably.

The lower on the scale of life one goes, the more dramatic are the results of fasting. The University of Chicago fasted an insect with a normal life span of only 24 hours. The insect lived for 15 days. A certain professor Huxley in England fasted one member of a family of planaria. That little fellow was still alive after 19 generations of his family had lived their lives and died.[11] Results are not this dramatic with higher organisms or human beings, but they are still significant.

JUICE OR WATER FASTING?

There is a great deal of debate over whether it is better to fast with just water or whether one should include juices or vegetable broths in the fast. European fasting clinics favor fasting with vegetable broths and juices in most instances. Many Americans favor water fasting.

Juice fasting assures plenty of liquid for washing away waste products. It is also valuable in helping to neutralize the acid condition of the tissues which is a result of fasting. Acidosis of fasting can result in muscle cramps.

Juice fasting is impossible when using the fast for detection of food allergy problems. A person might be allergic to the juice. Acidosis is dealt with in these situations by having patients breathe into a paper bag in some instances. This reverses the acidosis created by fasting.

Whichever form of fast a person might decide to undertake one warning should be given about juice fasting. Juice fasting or any other kind of imbalanced diet should not be continued for long periods of time. In one study it was actually found that dogs fed a demineralized diet survived only 26 to 30 days, while animals deprived of all food lived 40 to 60 days.[12]

BENEFITS OF A SHORT FAST

A frequently voiced concern is that a short fast may not have any health benefits. This is far from being true. A Dr. Bortz fasted rats for short periods of time and found that fasted rats outlived fattened cousins, almost doubling the normal life span. Fasted rats also refused to grow transplanted malignant tumors, while well-stuffed rats nurtured the transplanted tumors and died. Dr. Bortz concluded that most Americans would be better off if they ate half the food that they do now.[13] Dr. Alex Comfort found that mice not fed every third day had added fifty percent to their normal life span.[14]

Short fasts have also been found helpful in fighting disease. Going without food sharply increases the activity of the white blood cells in destroying disease germs in the body. In one study with rats the white blood cells of hungry animals had destroyed 4.23 bacteria for every white blood cell, while the white blood cells of well-fed animals had only destroyed 1.29 germs. The white blood cells did their best fighting 36 to 48 hours after fasting began. After 5 or 6 days this activity dwindled to almost nothing.[15]

SOME FASTING RECORDS

The longest controlled therapeutic fasting in medical history is probably a 249 day fast on juices and liquids at Stobhill General Hospital in Glasgow, Scotland. The patient was a 54 year old woman who lost 74 of her 262 pounds along with a painful arthritic knee condition.[16] Among the longest water fasts on record are those of nine of the companions of McSwiney, Lord Mayor of Cork, who fasted ninety-four days in 1920.[17]

It is not wise to try to set fasting records. There have been some serious problems develop among those who have undertaken long fasts. One popular magazine suggested that a prolonged fast of one hundred seventeen days contributed to gout in a three hundred and fifteen pound faster.[18]

A more scientific comment is made by two students of the subject who point out that there have been several deaths among fasting obese patients. However, in all but one case the deaths were apparently due to preexisting medical conditions aggravated by the obesity rather than by the fasting itself. The one exception was a 20 year old who in 30 weeks of fasting went from 260 pounds to 132 pounds. On the seventh day after she resumed eating her heartbeat became irregular and she died of ventricular fibrillation two days later. It was discovered that she had lost not only fat, but half of the lean tissue mass of her body during the fast.[19]

BREAKING THE FAST

By far the hardest part of fasting is breaking the fast. It is very difficult to control oneself when one begins eating again. This problem is beautifully illustrated by a little story Ted Mack shared about one of the unscheduled incidents on "The Original Amateur Hour." He told of how the dog star of an ill-fated commercial had been starved for three days so that he'd be sure to wolf down the dog food. He came on, gulped down the bowl of dog food, staggered about four paces and — live, in front of a TV audience of millions — upchucked the sponsor's product![20]

During a fast, cells have been found to shrink as much as 45 per cent.[21] After breaking the fast these altered cells have the ability to assimilate and utilize nutrients characteristic of the embryo or young person. In one case the tissues of a man of 40 were restored to the condition of a 17 year old after a 2 week fast.[22] Since what a person eats after fasting is very readily taken into the cells it is the course of prudence not to break a fast with mountains of junk food.

After a long fast there is a period of about two weeks during which a person tends to overeat. He should be watched or watch himself carefully during this period or he may damage himself.

It has long been the practice to break a fast with juices. Dr. Virginia Vetrano has recently demonstrated the superiority of breaking the fast with whole foods. This activates the salivary glands. It also reestablishes bowel function more rapidly than when a fast is broken with juices. When a fast is broken with juices a person has a stuffed feeling. This does not happen when a fast is broken with whole foods.[23]

FASTING AND CONTEMPORARY MEDICINE

Traditional medicine has not yet come to see the value of the old practice of fasting. Some modern pioneers of the medicine of the future have, however, found it an invaluable aid. Physicians have discovered that when they put patients on a five day fast the body clears itself of allergens (substances that the body has an allergic reaction to).

After a person has fasted for several days, foods are reintroduced into the diet one at a time. When the person eats a food he is allergic to or sensitive to the reaction is far stronger than it would normally be. Thus problem foods are easily detected and removed from the diet.

In other words, fasting is proving to be a valuable tool to help us listen to what our own bodies are telling us. Fasting may prove itself one of the most valuable tools available to us today. Physicians using this technique have already learned that allergies, diabetes and schizophrenia can often be dramatically improved.

Fasting is only a half-way solution, however. No fasting clinic separates the practice of fasting from good nutrition. Fasting was my first introduction to the field of nutrition. The first time I went to a fasting clinic I fasted. The second time I went to see how the people ate. I had become aware of the importance of nutrition. My interest in and love for nutrition was to grow as time went on.

CHAPTER 4

THE SYNERGISTIC EFFECT AND THE CHAIN OF LIFE

ONE of the most important things in life is relationships. A pillar of a certain girth and height may support a 500 pound weight beautifully. A thousand pound weight, on the other hand, might cause the very same pillar to splinter and disintegrate.

Relationships of substances or people can either facilitate the occurrence of a given event or retard the development of the phenomena involved. For example, an apple hanging on a tree tends to fall to the earth. If the apple falls on some twigs and branches that have tightly grown together, it may never reach the earth. We would say that the twigs were antagonistic to the occurrence of the falling of the apple.

On the other hand, there are often ways in which things work together. This is what is meant by the synergistic effect. There are many things that could speed the falling of the apple. A windy day might dislodge the apple from its stem. Lack of water or a warm summer day might hurry the ripening of the apple. A bird might dislodge the apple while trying to eat it, or a human hand might pluck the apple. All of these are examples of the "synergistic effect."

NUTRIENTS WORK TOGETHER

The synergistic effect is very important for an understanding of nutrition, because all nutrients work together. For example, a number of years ago it was discovered that children suffering from kwashiorkor (medically defined as a protein deficiency disease) did not respond when given a high grade protein supplement (powdered skim milk). Another group of doctors, however, treating eye diseases of the children with vitamin A were startled to see the signs of protein deficiency clearing up.[1]

Other nutrients are necessary for the use of protein in the diet. One of the eight essential building blocks of protein, methionine, can not be properly handled when vitamin B6 is inadequately supplied in the diet.[2]

Adequate use of protein is also dependent upon the ability of the body to break it down in the stomach and intestines. A lack of hydrochloric acid, the acid produced in the stomach that helps us digest our food, will result in very poor use of protein. A lack of B1, B2, B3, B6, choline and folic acid can detrimentally affect hydrochloric acid (HCL) production.[3] Glutamic acid, one of the amino acids, is of particular importance for HCL production. Thus a deficiency of glutamic acid can result in a deficiency of HCL. Without HCL, glutamic acid is poorly used, perpetuating the HCL deficiency. A lack of HCL will also result in mineral deficiencies.

The cement which binds tissues together is composed of protein and vitamin C. In healthy tissue this cement looks like clear jelly streaked with darker bands of greater strength, like reinforcing rods in concrete. When vitamin C is inadequate, the tissue cement becomes more liquid and cells pull apart. Actually, this is what scurvy is — a person literally comes unglued![4]

You will remember the importance of vitamin A for the ability of the body to use protein. Zinc is critical for the ability of the body to use vitamin A. Vitamin A is stored in the liver and zinc is necessary for its release.

Zinc and copper are both important for the formation of connective tissue. Lack of these nutrients can result in stretch marks in the skin or other tissues. Vitamin B6 is also involved in the formation of connective tissue.[5]

Vitamin A is poorly absorbed if there is inadequate unsaturated fat in the diet. Diabetics do not metabolize fats well and thus run a special risk of developing vitamin A deficiency.

What is the point of all this? The reactions which have been discussed simply indicate the different nutrients required by the body to properly use protein, and this discussion has only been fragmentary. It becomes a critical point in one's understanding of nutrition to realize that all nutrients work together.

It is fine to study nutrients in isolation — that is how we find out what they do — but it is the height of foolishness to try to nourish oneself with only isolated nutrients. Unfortunately, this is the trap we have fallen into. We remove twenty five or so nutrients from our bread and add back large amounts of five or six and call the bread enriched. Many people supplement their diets with vitamins and minerals in the same way that they eat — in a very fragmented and partial way.

THE CHAIN OF LIFE

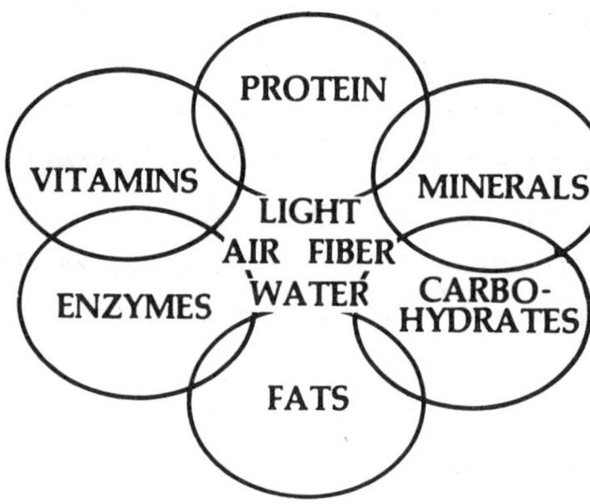

The expression "the chain of life" refers to the nutritive substances necessary for the life of the cells of the body. These substances enable the body to derive energy from the food we eat or provide the energy the cells need.

The illustration of the chain was chosen by Roger Williams to emphasize the fact that all links in the chain are needed by the body. Nutrition is only as strong as its weakest link. Because of the synergistic effect with which nutrients work with one another, when one link is missing the entire chain is weakened, destroying what would otherwise be a very favorable environment for the life of the cells. Each link in the chain of life meets a special need. No one nutrient can do the work of another.[6]

The preceding diagram in this chapter shows only the major categories of nutrients known to be important for health. To deal with all the 60 or 70 odd nutrients now known to be important for good health individually is a subject for a book itself.

All the individual links in the chain of life are necessary for maintaining the machinery of the body and keeping things going. However, one part of the body frequently needs one link in the chain more than another. For example, the thyroid gland is far more dependent upon iodine than most other tissues. If this nutrient is not supplied to this part of the body, goiter will result. The eye and epithelial tissues are dependent upon vitamin A. The blood needs iron for its hemoglobin. The lungs need zinc for the release of carbon dioxide. This means, as was explained in the last chapter, that while the lack of a particular nutrient will be detrimental to the whole body, its lack will often affect one part of the body more than another.

The list of items in the nutritional chain of life as far as the particulars is always changing. Nutrition is a relatively young and growing science. As of now there are about 60 nutrients which are felt to be important for health. Eventually there could be as many as 100. The list of important nutritional substances could eventually be much greater than even this.

The key to obtaining all of these diverse substances important for the life of the cells is to eat food from many different sources. It is rare in nature to find a food which has even most of the nutrients now recognized to be of importance for good health. Lack or shortage of any item will result in ill health and eventually in death.

Consumption of every nutrient at every meal is not necessary. The body does have the ability to store nutrients. Reserves for some nutrients can be quite large, while other nutrients are poorly stored by the body. For example, oil soluble vitamins are well stored by the body, while water soluble vitamins are stored only with great difficulty by the body. When these reserves are depleted life functions begin to be hampered.

There are many particulars in the chain of life, but the following section looks at the larger categories.

PROTEIN

The word protein is derived from the Greek language and means "to come first." Protein is of first importance as far as health is concerned. The body can use protein in place of fat or carbohydrate, but there is no way in which the body can convert fat or carbohydrate to protein for use in constructing healthy tissues. Fat and carbohydrate are energy foods. Protein can also be used for energy by the body, but it is far more important for building new tissue or repairing damage in the body.

When a person looks in the mirror much of what is seen is protein. It is a major constituent of skin, hair, and fingernails. Inadequate protein intake or poor use of this nutrient can result in hair loss, sagging skin, and brittle fingernails that break or chip easily.

The inside of the body is partially composed of protein. This includes organs such as the heart, lungs, nervous system and brain. The enzymes that aid in digestion of food contain protein as do the hormones that control much of the body chemistry. Protein is also important for the formation of antibodies which aid in resistance to disease.

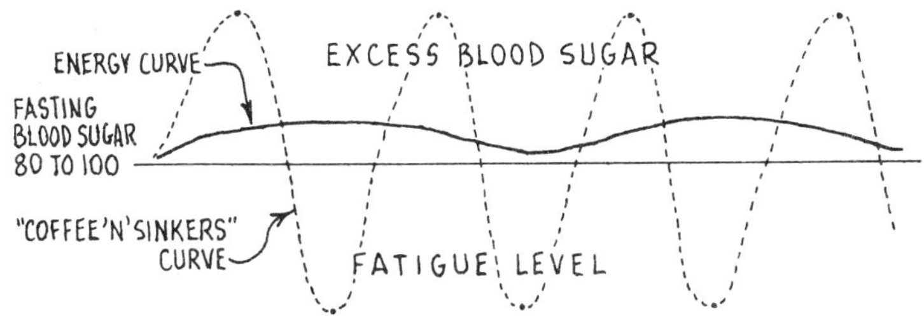

THE COFFEE AND SINKERS CURVE

Blood sugar provides nourishment for the muscles, brain and nerves. When blood sugar is stable the body operates at a peak of efficiency. When blood sugar levels become erratic, a person experiences fatigue, inability to think and nervous irritability. "Coffee and Sinkers" refers to coffee and doughnuts. The combination of caffeine (which releases stored sugar from the liver into the blood) and sugar (which is readily absorbed into the bloodstream) can disturb blood sugar levels, by creating a very rapid rise in blood sugar followed by a sudden plunge. Complex carbohydrate and protein foods help to stabilize blood sugar by a slow and consistent release of sugar or "glucose" into the blood.

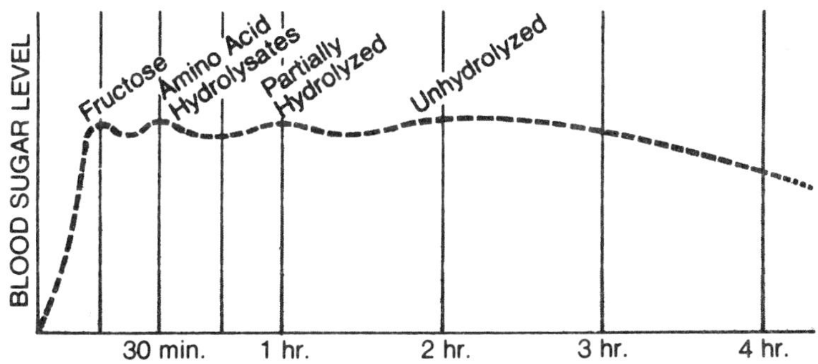

A TIMED ENERGY RELEASE PROTEIN SUPPLEMENT

This is an example of the way in which one protein supplement was manufactured in order to supply a longer energy curve and a more stable blood sugar. Ingredients with different degrees of availability were mixed. Fructose (fruit sugar) was added for instant energy. Highly hydrolyzed proteins are added for backup energy. (Hydro = water and lysis = to loose). The bonds of a protein are "loosed" or digested by the addition of water between the bonds. This is why protein can be dehydrating if a person's fluid intake is inadequate. Partially hydrolyzed (or broken apart) protein and unhydrolyzed protein provide sustained high blood sugar levels.

THE EIGHT ESSENTIAL AMINO ACIDS *

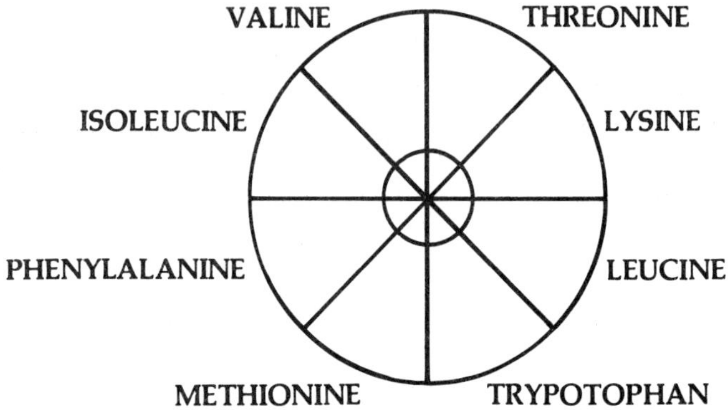

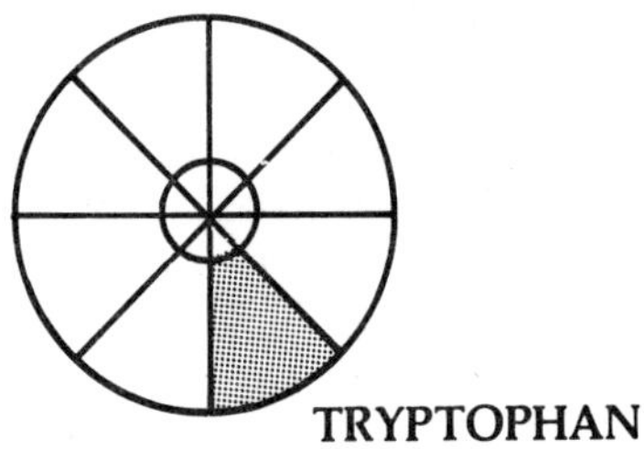

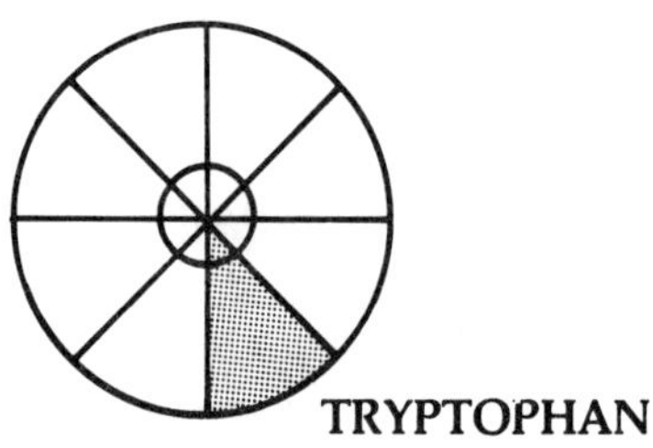

**Histidine and argenine are necessary for growth in children. Thus children have ten essential amino acids.*

BALANCE

When one of the essential building blocks (amino acids) of protein is partially missing in the diet the body can only partially use the others. When one of the essential amino acids is completely missing the ability of the body to use the protein at all comes into question.

←

PARTIAL LACK OF AN AMINO ACID

←

Corn is inadequately supplied with trypotophan, a fact partially responsible for the widespread incidence of pellagra (vitamin B3 deficiency) in the southern United States during the early years of the 20th century.

The body can convert tryptophan into niacin, a bonus in view of the difficulty of obtaining adequate niacin in the diet from the food we eat.

TOTAL LACK OF AN AMINO ACID

←

Gelatin is 100% protein, but because it lacks the essential amino acid tryptophan, it is of little value as a biological source of protein when eaten by itself.

Some Yardsticks for Protein Quality

One yardstick for protein quality is *balance*. Protein is composed of building blocks called amino acids. These are important for the construction of protein by the body, just as the letters of the alphabet are essential for the construction of words.[7]

Eight of the amino acids are called "essential". This means that the body can not build protein without these essential building blocks. Scientists have learned that all these building blocks must be present at the same meal in adequate quantities to be used to build protein.

Many protein foods are partially or totally lacking in one or more of the essential building blocks. Gelatin, a favorite remedy for brittle fingernails, is lacking in the amino acid known as tryptophan. Gelatin consumed by itself is therefore of little value for helping fingernails or any other tissue suffering from lack of protein.

Corn is partially lacking in the same amino acid, tryptophan. This decreases its value as a protein food. Protein foods are unbalanced by cooking because some amino acids are destroyed or rendered unusable to the body by heat. Balance of the amino acids in a protein is without a doubt a yardstick of quality.

A second yardstick of the quality of a protein involves a process called *denaturing*. High levels of heat change some proteins, altering their basic nature.[8] The higher the heat the greater the risk of altering the characteristics of the protein.

Most people are quite familiar with how a protein is denatured. Almost everyone has observed that they can drop a raw egg in a blender and blend it with water. Try that trick with a fried egg, however. It simply will not work. The egg has been changed from a water-loving (hydrophylic) to a water-fearing (hydrophobic) substance. The nature of the protein has been changed.

The less heat applied to protein foods, the less chance

of their being denatured. Cooking is sometimes necessary, however, to destroy potential parasites in some meats in particular. The potential health damage that could result from consuming overly heated foods has not yet been thoroughly investigated. Dr. Francis Pottenger did feed cats cooked foods from one generation to another and documented a deterioration in their health which was staggering.[9]

A third yardstick for the quality of a protein is its *digestability*. Many protein foods are difficult to digest and can actually wear out the enzyme systems of the body in attempting to digest them. Legumes such as peanuts and soybeans can be difficult to digest, as can large quantities of meat. Overcooking a protein food can make it more difficult to digest.

When problems with the digestion of protein foods develop, the person can choose foods which are easier to digest. Yogurt, for example, is easier to digest than is milk. Fish is usually easier on the digestive tract than red meat. Supplementation with hydrochloric acid and pancreatic enzymes may be necessary in extreme cases of indigestion.

The Protective Function of Protein

Many people develop a craving or addiction for sweets. Some have suggested that this craving is a result of starvation of the pituitary gland for protein. Adequate protein intake does frequently help to curb the appetite for sweets.

Dr. Arthur Furst, one of the foremost nutritional researchers in the United States, did considerable work for the national space program. One of the problems he dealt with was the reprocessing of waste products for consumption during long term space flights. In the reprocessing he wound up with refined carbohydrates. When he fed these to laboratory rats, the rats died.

When Dr. Furst fed his animals supplemental protein with the refined carbohydrates the animals were protected.

Dr. John Yudkin conducted a similar experiment. He fed laboratory rats high levels of sugar with low protein content in the diet. The rats became nearsighted. When rats were fed supplemental protein along with a high sugar intake their eyes were not affected. Refined carbohydrates increase the requirement for protein in the diet. Rats fed only marginally adequate protein suffer a setback in growth when sugar is added to the diet. Sugar reduces the ability of the body to utilize protein in these circumstances.[10] Protein appears to be able to protect the body from some of the harmful effects of sugar consumption if adequately supplied in the diet — an important point when one realizes that millions of American teenagers eat a low protein-high sugar diet.

ESSENTIAL FATS

High quality fats are very important for good health, but they have been whisked out of the American diet with a magician's sleight of hand. The high quality fats frequently undersupplied in the American diet have been called the essential fatty acids (lipids and sterols). Their function and importance are discussed in another chapter.

When the essential fats are exposed to oxygen or heat they spoil rapidly and ruin the taste and smell of food. This happens whenever a nut is shelled or a grain of wheat is cracked. Wheat germ left exposed to the air will turn rancid in about two weeks from the time it is separated from the grain. Many people who use wheat germ have never tasted a fresh product.

Because of the ease with which natural oils turn rancid, the food industry has developed methods for processing grains and oils to remove these fats. This is why we have white bread, white rice, and filtered oils. Such processing greatly increases the storage life of foods but decreases their nutritional value.

Nuts and butter are high oil foods that can easily turn rancid. Sometimes these foods are heavily salted to cover a rancid or "off" taste. Fresh foods are superior to both processed foods with oils removed and to food with rancid oils from the standpoint of taste and nutritional value.

VITAMINS

One will not find long discussions of individual vitamins in this chapter nor in this book. The reason for this is that vitamins work in complexes. From the standpoint of all around nutrition it only makes sense to obtain complexes of all the vitamins and minerals in the diet, rather than trying to rely on one or two nutrients.

Vitamins are the spark plugs of the system. They are catalysts that facilitate the reactions going on in the body. Most of the activities carried out by the body involve large numbers of different nutrients.

Where nutrition is complete very small quantities of vitamins are needed by the body. Where severe malnutrition exists in a person's past, an acquired need for larger than normal amounts of nutrients can develop. This has been demonstrated to occur among former Japanese prisoners of war with vitamin B3.[11]

Sometimes we do not really appreciate the importance of vitamins because we hear so much about them. This is due to a poor sense of history. Millions of people have suffered and died throughout the course of history duc to lack of one vitamin or another. The problem has become much more serious with the advent of processed foods. Even before this, however, scurvy killed multitudes in Europe for centuries. Beri-beri (vitamin B1 deficiency) annihilated the Japanese navy for years, and pellagra (vitamin B3 deficiency) spread a dark shroud of misery over the southern United States for years.

The discovery of nutrition was no accident and no outgrowth of idle curiosity. Each and every stage in the discovery of nutrition was an outgrowth of a crying need.

Widespread nutritional deficiencies began to develop in human beings when they left warmer climates. Rickets (vitamin D deficiency) developed among people in northern climates with inadequate exposure to light. Scurvy developed where people could not grow fresh foods during the wintertime. Soil erosion, due to poor farming practices, depleted crops of trace minerals and protein.

When food processing was introduced it created further deficiencies. Sugar and other refined foods robbed the body of the essential B vitamins. Consumption of one main food (corn) led to widespread vitamin B3 deficiencies.

Thus as poor dietary habits and environmental changes led to widespread deficiencies, nutritional needs became apparent. The door to the discovery of the science of nutrition was born.

MINERALS

Vitamins need minerals to properly perform their work. Many minerals are needed by the body in such minute quantities that their importance was overlooked until quite recently. Trace mineral nutrition has proven itself extraordinarily complex and also very important.

The trace mineral selenium illustrates the care with which trace mineral nutrition must be handled. Inadequate intake of selenium has been shown to increase the risk of cancer. Excess selenium can produce death. The difference between the two levels is not a very large one.

It has been suggested that the extraordinarily long lives of some people in the world is a result of a particularly fortuitous combination of minerals in their drinking water. The water these people drink is heavily silted, meaning that it is rich in minerals.[12]

The teeth are a reflection of the overall fitness of the body. Minerals are, of course, very important for good teeth. Dr. Weston Price found that people consuming large quantities of fish had fewer dental caries than people on any other diet that he examined.[13] Fish contain not only a high quality of protein, but also large quantities of trace minerals. Natural sources of vitamins with associated trace minerals include cod and other fish liver oils (vitamin A complex), yeast concentrates (vitamin B complex), citrus and pepper (red and green) concentrates, (vitamin C complex), wheat germ concentrates (vitamin E complex), dessicated liver (vitamin B complex) and kelp (trace minerals).

CARBOHYDRATES

Carbohydrates provide the body with the fuel on which it can operate. Complex, unrefined carbohydrates provide the body with a stable energy source. Refined carbohydrates such as sugar and white flour are more difficult for the body to properly metabolize. Imbalances are set up in the system, which can lead to health problems.

A natural component of a complex carbohydrate food is fiber. When foods are processed or cooked, the fiber is broken down. Fiber normalizes the operation of the digestive tract and aids the body in the proper handling of fat. Lack of fiber can result in the breakdown of bile (a digestive substance produced by the liver) into cancer causing compounds in the colon.[14]

SUMMARY

The body needs all the nutrients in the different categories discussed above. Lack of one nutrient can throw a monkey wrench into the operation of the body as a whole. The best argument in favor of complete nutrition is the fact that all nutrients work together, what we have called "the synergistic effect".

Complete nutrition consists of the "chain of life." The goal of sound nutrition can be met by striving to eat the foods and take the food supplements which will provide all the nutrients in the chain of life. Food supplementation which aims to adequately provide the chain of life should include not only vitamins and minerals but also quality sources of enzymes, protein and the essential fatty acids (lipids and sterols). Adequate exposure to sunlight and fresh air and consumption of pure water and indigestable fiber should round out the nutritional picture.

CHAPTER 5

FOUR FACTOR NUTRITION SHE WALKED AGAIN

I volunteered to help my parents with their nutrition business after my father became involved in a chemical fire and suffered severe lung damage. A short while later I found myself at a convention talking with a little lady with an amazing story. We sat in the hotel lobby.

The little lady's eyes sparkled as she looked at me. She was the first person I talked to at the convention. "How did you become involved with nutrition?" I asked.

She began to tell her story. "I was working as an RN when I suffered a hip and back injury while trying to get a heavy patient up in bed. After a few weeks, arthritis set in my hip. I was put in traction in the hospital two different times for a total of 29 days. I was in the hospital three months. My right hip was injected with large amounts of cortisone while I was in traction and after I left the hospital."

"I was given 100 capsules of butizolidin before I went to the hospital. This was to relax the tendons torn loose in my right groin. This caused all my joints to become so relaxed that they all got so they slid around when I moved and I had no control of them."

She leaned forward dramatically, joining her thumb and index finger in front of my face. "It was so bad," she said, "that my joints would slip out when I picked up a piece of paper. I could tip over at my knees forwards, or sideways the same as backwards. I could not stand."

I was sent to San Francisco three times to visit bone specialists. Nothing could be done for me. Five days of tests proved negative. My only discernable problems were arthritis in the hip, edema in the legs, and an inability to control the joints due to the medications and perhaps partially due to traction. I was suffering from severe pain and was sent home from San Francisco with *permanent disability.*

"After returning home to Eureka I was sent to a bone specialist again." He said, "Well, you are in pretty bad shape, aren't you!" I replied "Well, it looks like it." He repeated, "Well, you are in pretty bad shape", and added, "Well, you are on your own now." I said "I'm on my own now?" and he said, "Yes, you are on your own now!"

"We went home and started doing everything natural. I went off all medication. My husband had to lift me in and out of bed, turn me from side to side, undress and dress me, comb my hair, lift me in and out of the wheel chair, etc. When being moved I would cry and yell with pain in spite of myself. My son thought I should have my leg cut off so I wouldn't suffer so. I was ready to die."

"My wonderful husband fed me raw vegetable juices, vitamins and minerals. That didn't do the trick. I did improve, but was still unable to walk. The elders of the church were gathered together and offered special prayer for me."

"God did not see fit to heal me at that time. Finally, I prayed that God would lead me to find something that would heal my body so that I would be able to walk again."

"My husband was selling soap at that time, and one of the men in a meeting only a very short time after that prayer, was a food supplement distributor. He told us about four factor supplementation. After using complete supplements only four months I was able to walk by myself, I have continually improved since that time."

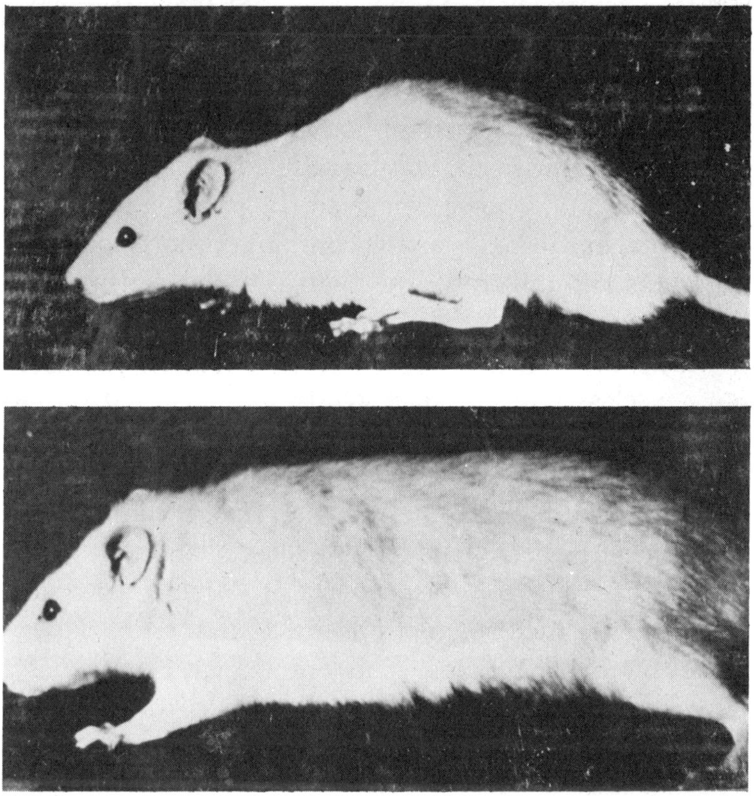

The two rats shown were twins. The one on top was fed a normal rat ration. The one on the bottom was fed the same ration with the addition of a four factor supplement which contained vitamins, minerals, protein and essential fatty acids obtained from grain concentrates. Autopsy revealed that the animal given complete supplementation was experiencing better health, but this much is obvious just from a casual glance at the two animals. Nutrition is rarely optimal in nature.

A VISIT TO A MEDICAL CONVENTION

I was still pondering the question of why vitamins and minerals had not helped this lady as I boarded the plane. The head of the firm I was travelling with showed me a photograph of a horse before and after being fed a fundamental nutritional ration containing more than just vitamins and minerals. The change in the health of the animal was remarkable. The first horse looked like a relic of the Civil War, a wreck ready for the glue factory, or a useless bag of bones ready to be turned out to pasture. The second photograph showed a horse vibrant with health, ready to be placed on the race track and to hold his head high. Could nutrition make that kind of a difference? It seemed almost unbelievable to me.

The occasion for this trip was to attend a medical convention. Such conventions are an interesting experience for the uninitiated. This one was in Kansas City. Speakers were gathered from all parts of the country. Lectures were given in several small rooms.

A large ballroom was filled with booths. Pharmacutical companies displayed their products at these booths. Manufacturer's representatives manned them. I was amazed at the scope of the various products displayed.

As I wandered those isles I came upon a relization as powerful as any of the points made by the speakers that week. Many of the booths contained hormones or glandular concentrates of one kind or another. The numbers and varieties of these substances boggled my mind. Numerous books, pamphlets and handouts on hormones were also there.

I realized that these physicians had to deal with endocrine problems on a day to day basis. There would not have been so many of these products if the doctors did not feel the need for them in their practice.

I had studied the hormones and what they did for the

body previously, but had felt that problems of hormone or glandular imbalance were relatively infrequent and therefore of little significance. Now I began to rethink what I had learned.

Most of the things I saw at this convention were in line with what I had learned about the history of hormone development.

THE DANGER OF STRESS

Stress has the ability to warp, maim, and even kill an individual.

Psychologist F. G. Zimbardo feels that packing people together in large cities alters a person's frame of mind creating a submerged vindictiveness. He sought to demonstrate this by parking an automobile on a street in two locations.

One automobile he parked on a street in lower Manhattan near New York University. Another automobile was parked on a street in a much smaller city, Palo Alto, near Stanford University.

In each case Zimbardo selected middle class neighborhoods near these universities. He left the hoods of the cars up to indicate mechanical trouble, and then retreated behind a nearby window to observe.

In New York City it took just seven minutes for vandalism to set in, and by the time sixty-four hours had passed, the car was a "battered, useless hunk of metal, the result of twenty-three incidents of destructive contact." Most of the culprits worked by daylight, and were well-dressed, white, middle-class adults.

By contrast the car parked in pleasant Palo Alto went unharmed, although not untouched. When rain began to fall a kindly pedestrian stopped and lowered the hood to keep the motor dry.[1]

NOT ALL STRESS IS BAD

The harmful effects of stress are almost proverbial in our thinking, but this concept is really quite incorrect. Stress can also be very beneficial. It prevents boredom and keeps a person moving and alive.

There is a story about herring fishermen off the coast of England. Herring are a very sensitive fish and seem to know when they are prisoners. When they were dumped into huge tanks on the deck of fishing ships they would stop swimming, turn sluggish and lose color and freshness.

One clever captain developed a strategy for keeping his herring fresh and lively right to the dock. He put one catfish in each tank! The catfish loves herring for dinner, so this one lone catfish chased after the herring all the way to the dock, keeping them moving and fresh. Though the catfish ate a few herring, the rest brought a much better price at the market.[2]

Some people need more stress than others, but we all need some stress in order to challenge us and bring out our best capabilities. Stress can be created when life is too easy as well as when it is too hard. If this were not so, many businessmen would not die shortly after retirement. They die because of the stresses of boredom!

The fact that an easy life relatively free from stresses and difficulty can shorten lifespan has been demonstrated in the laboratory. A study of over a thousand animals showed that those subjected to cares and joys, setbacks and surprises of every kind lived longer and were more immune to illness than those who were kept under "ideal conditions."[3]

A person's requirements for stress and ability to handle it are dependent upon his own unique makeup. Some people are lions and need the excitement of the stalking of prey, the wild rush of attack, and the savage battle and triumphant kill.

Other people are like the crocodile and need to live life in a little more tranquil way. A lion could never be happy lying in the mud all day, nor could the crocodile be happy trying to live the life of a lion.[4]

Each person must and is probably naturally inclined to find his or her own stress level. We need to run at our own pace and in pursuit of those things which we desire.

Some people need to live at the pace of a turtle. Others are able to maintain the pace of the proverbial hare. Despite the familiarity of the fable in which the turtle outraces the hare, the surest way for a turtle to kill himself is to feel that he must live like a rabbit.

Each person must pursue his own direction in life. Some people naturally are happy with things. Others need to be around people to be truly happy. Some people are motivated by money while others could care less. A life direction should be chosen which results in satisfaction.

Not all stress is unpleasant. Some stress is quite pleasant. A young couple in a passionate embrace is a good example of stress — but it is a pleasant stress.

HANDLING STRESS

Stress needs to be confronted forthrightly and dealt with realistically. Running away from stress rarely resolves problems. One dying cowboy shared the greatest lesson he ever learned on the prairies as follows:

> The Herefords taught me one of life's most important lessons. We used to breed cattle for a living but the severe winter storms used to take an awful toll. Again and again after a severe winter storm we would find most of them piled up against fences dead. They would turn their backs to the icy blasts and slowly drift down wind twenty miles until the fence stopped them. There they piled up and died.

> The Herefords were different. They would head straight into the wind and slowly work up the other way until they came to our upper boundary fence where they stood facing into the storm. We always found them alive and well. That's the greatest lesson I ever learned on the prairies.[5]

The secret of handling stress is to know when and to what extent to defend oneself. Sometimes it is the course of prudence not to use one's ability to defend oneself. The body does not need to call on an all out defense against a mosquito bite. On the other hand, if defense is inadequate in the presence of a cancer cell, death will result.

Just as this principle of appropriateness of response to stressing agents is true on the cellular level, so is it true on the level of the individual. Over reacting to very small stresses is something seen almost daily. You also may be familiar with situations in which a father gives not only an ulcer to himself, but also donates one to the rest of the family because they are going to be late to dinner. A glass of spilled milk can give some people an ulcer, though it should not.

Emotions are not improper if they aid in resolving stress, but if they magnify stress they can be very dangerous and harmful. Screaming at one's child for spilling a glass of milk accidentally is a worthless and unnecessary use of emotion. If the spilling of the milk is purposeful, then an appropriate display of anger may be worthwhile.

Over reacting to a stressor may do more harm to us than it does to the object or person attacked. John Hunter, a great physiologist, once said, "The first scoundrel that gets me angry will kill me." Later at a medical meeting a speaker made comments that angered Hunter. As he stood up and bitterly attacked the speaker, his anger affected his heart and he fell over dead.[6]

The greatest danger not only to the individual, but to the world today is over reacting to small irritations. On the world scene small incidents can conceivably result in nuclear war if nations over react. One hopes that the nations of the world will have a better record on this than we do as individuals.

A HISTORY OF STRESS RESEARCH

The man who pioneered stress research was Hans Selye, an Austrian born endocrinologist. He did much of his work at a large set of research laboratories at the University of Montreal.

In 1926 as a second year medical student Selye first observed that there appeared to be common factors to many diverse ailments. Sick people, even to a green medical student, looked sick. His professors were only observing the differences in patients and not looking at the similarities.

By 1936 Selye had established himself in Montreal. In working with laboratory rats he noted that the rats reacted the same internally, no matter what kind of stressor they were subject to. He also noted that the adrenal gland was the body's prime responder to stress.

The adrenal glands are the only part of the body that thrive and enlarge under stress. Other organs shrink and hemorrhage under stress. Selye also discovered that he could induce many degenerative diseases by subjecting his laboratory animals to high levels of stress.

At length Selye arrived at a definition for stress: STRESS IS THE NONSPECIFIC RESPONSE OF THE BODY TO ANY DEMAND.[7] Stress is a drastic wearing force. Each person has a different hereditary capacity to withstand stress, but once this capacity or "adaptation energy" has been expended it cannot be replenished. It is like a nation's deposits of oil. Once the oil has been removed from the ground and burned it is gone forever.[8]

Selye discovered that certain substances called hormones were key in the ability of the body to respond to stress. The most important hormones were those of the adrenal gland (shaped like a tiny pancake on top of the kidneys) and the pituitary gland hormones (this gland is about the size of a pea and is located in the very center of the brain).

Hormones control the overall functioning of the body. When their balance is upset through some kind of stressor the overall functioning of the body is affected. Selye called the response of the body to a stressor the "General Adaptation Syndrome."

THE GENERAL ADAPTATION SYNDROME

This term refers to the generalized response of the body to any sudden change in the environment. There are three phases to the body's response to stressors. These are the *alarm reaction,* the *stage of resistance,* and the *stage of exhaustion.*

The *alarm reaction* is a drastic response of the body to any sudden change in the environment. A sudden loud noise is a good example. Almost any sudden loud noise will cause an alarm reaction in human beings. Our bodies have not learned to distinguish the honking of the horn of a rude motorist from the trumpeting challenge of some wild beast. This is unfortunate because in our noise polluted society we are constantly being stressed.

The *alarm reaction* has drastic effects upon the body. The adrenal gland is the body's key responder to stress. It doubles in size when the body is stressed and changes color from a whitish-yellow to a reddish-brown. This is because a whitish lipid or fatty coating of the gland is utilized during stress in the production of anti-stress hormones.

There is intense tissue breakdown when the body is stressed. The thymus, a key to resisting disease, withers away. The stomach lining becomes spotted with bleeding ulcers. Growth and sex cease.

One of the interesting facets of the alarm reaction to stress is the withdrawal of blood from the extremities. It has been suggested that this reaction is a natural defensive posture on the part of the body.

In nature, stress is frequently followed by a physical attack. The arm will not bleed as seriously if blood is withdrawn from the extremities as if the blood remained there. Blood pressure rises under stress as well, due to the constriction of circulation when it is withdrawn from the extremities.

The second phase of response to stress is the *stage of resistance.* This is observed by placing animals or humans in contact with a prolonged stress. The body appears to return to normal in this stage.

The adrenal glands refill empty stores with lipids and revert to normal size. The thymus regains its mass. Body chemistry, seriously imbalanced during the alarm reaction, returns to normal. In this stage the animal's resistance to the initial stressor is increased. Unfortunately, resistance to any other stressor is decreased. For example, a person might be able to resist the loud noise of living close to an airport, but as a consequence have decreased resistance to the flu virus.

The third phase of response to stress is the *stage of exhaustion.* This takes place when the stress is prolonged beyond the ability of the body to endure it or nutritional reserves are inadequate to foster resistance. All defenses collapse and life eventually ceases. One of the hallmarks of this period is the development of degenerative diseases which we ordinarily think of as the "old age" diseases of man.

Degenerative diseases can be produced in very young people if they are subjected to enough stress. These might include hypertension, cardiovascular disease, gastro-intestinal disorders, allergies, mental disease or arthritis. The onset of these problems is usually preceeded by an extended period of chronic fatigue, for which this stage of response to stress is named.[9]

DISCOVERY OF HORMONES

Dr. Selye's work led to the introduction of hormone therapy to medicine.

A group of medical men met in Chicago in 1949 to report on the first attempts to deal with hormone imbalances by using recently developed ACTH (pituitary hormone) and cortisone.

One physician at the meeting reported, "Never have I attended such a conference. It was like a religious meeting, with men popping up all over the house to tell of some seeming miracle.

No medical gathering in history ever heard reports of so many different diseases yielding to treatment with a single drug. Acute asthma, pneumonia, chronic alcholism, rheumatic fever — diseases described in the medical books as widely contrasting disorders, each with its own pattern of symptons — had all been mastered, at least during treatment . . ."[10]

Walter Bauer of the Harvard University Medical School said, "the astonishing ability of ACTH apparently to turn diseases off and on at will marks the opening of a new era in medicine." J.S.L. Browne said, "The emotional impact of that Chicago conference was terrific. As disease after disease was reported on, I sat enthralled, feeling that we were witnessing the beginning of a revolution."[11] Another commented, "Even cancer, in some forms (leukemia), seems to yield temporarily to the influence of ACTH."[12]

With all of this early enthusiasm one wonders what happened, as hormones are used very cautiously today.

It was soon discovered that the results of injecting hormones are often unpredictable.

For example, ACTH may stop acute attacks of gout, but when administered in a quiet period between attacks can bring on an upflare of the disease. Side effects of using these hormones included heightened blood pressure, severe headaches, edema, excessive hair growth, skin eruptions and occasional confused mental states.[13]

Since this time many competent physicians have become wary of cortisone, feeling that used in the quantities needed to get results it upsets the balances of different body hormones. Protracted use of cortisone can also result in adrenal atrophy.

These physicians frequently use injections of an extract of beef adrenals which contains the whole assortment of adrenal hormones in the balance drawn up by nature. This extract enables the exhausted adrenal glands of a patient to crawl into bed and rest while the added hormones take over and do the work.

NUTRITION AND STRESS

In 1946 a group of research workers at Hollywood Presbyterian Hospital in Los Angeles began a series of studies on coping with stress and hormone imbalances through nutrition. This approach was a sharp departure from the path being taken by the majority of the medical profession. The researchers sought to find out why people were breaking down under the stresses we experience today. They figured that part of the problem was with our food which has been continually "refined" and "purified" since 1900.

Since this food is made available through the body chemistry they felt that this must be part of the problem. The chemistry of the body is controlled through the endocrine glands and the hormones they secrete so they chose to begin their study here.

The technology for analyzing the urine for the presence of hormones had just become available. The goal of research was to determine if urinary residue of hormones accurately reflects hormonal sufficiency in supply and function in the living body. Study began with 60 patients in a large sanitarium.

The results of the initial study indicated consistent aberrations in several basic health-maintaining functions. The body was not producing adequate amounts of hormones to balance body chemistry. The researchers did not figure that giving hormones by injection was the answer since these are seized as rapidly as possible by the liver and inactivated.

The common sense of the researchers told them that the body was designed to produce hormones in a balanced and adequate way. They felt that somewhere in nature were the substances the body could use to develop its own hormones.

After much trial and error it was found that minute quantities of these substances were found in the whole grains. These substances were concentrated in the form of a supplement, using wheat, rice and soybean extracts.[14]

Results of supplementation of the diet of hospital patients with vitamins, minerals, protein, and these grain concentrates were quite significant from two standpoints. Firstly, there was sometimes dramatic improvement in chronic degenerative conditions. Secondly, there was often overall improvement in the balance of body chemistry as measured by hormone residue in the urine.

One woman who had been a rheumatoid arthritic for 8 years experienced dramatic improvement. She could not stand the sheets on her feet at night, and could not pick up a dish. She could not get comfortable in bed at night, but would get up and pace the floor.

Many conventional medical treatments for the problem had been tried including ACTH, cortisone, salycilated sodium, and aspirin. None had helped. She noticed an improvement within 10 days of supplementing the diet and made gradual improvement. Her husband was so impressed by this improvement that when the medical research on this food supplement was completed after a 12 year period he bought the formula and began a food supplement company.

FOUR FACTOR SUPPLEMENTATION

The orchestration or coordination of body functions is carried out by the hormones and nervous system. The development of this four-factor supplement (vitamins, minerals, protein, and lipids) appeared to have improved overall body function with hospital patients. The researchers were curious as to whether this kind of supplementation would be beneficial for the average American. They decided to carry on some studies with athletes, the healthiest portion of the population and that portion of the population most in contrast with the patients in the hospital which had been the subjects of study.

The following is a summary of the number of competent metabolisms found among various groups of athletes when biochemical testing was done:

Group	Protein Regeneration	Energy Output	Acid Base Balance	Vitamins Minerals Utilization
High School Boys (80)	1	0	0	0
College Men (210)	0	3	0	0
Pro-football (310)	4	11	0	1
Muscle Builders (70)	6	0	7	0
Controls (18)	2	2	5	3

The above figures were arrived at in a rather interesting test. The athletes were first tested on the morning before games and then on the morning after. It was these post-game tests 18 hours after competition which showed competitors to be measurably down in overall reserves in all the tests.

Pre-game condition was found to be apparently adequate. This means that these better-than average human beings carried just enough reserve biological vigor to meet one stress crisis in an adequate way. If another stress had quickly followed the results might have been disastrous.

This test with athletes was designed to show what happens to individuals who are apparently above the norm in health when given two forms of supplementation of the diet. Controls were given a three factor supplement with vitamins, minerals, and protein, while all other groups were given a four factor supplement with vitamins, minerals, protein, and the essential lipids.

The controls felt more energetic with the supplements, many of them "raring to go." Biochemical testing, however, showed that they were making no improvement as far as the 4 basic tests. They lacked the definitive factor in meeting stress: endurance. This was due to their poor performance in the basic biological functions being tested.

Among athletes given the four factor supplement a distincition due to age was obvious almost from the start. Younger men showed definitive results in biochemical testing and on the playing field within two months. They had endurance and fighting heart.

Older athletes experienced a three-month time lag before they also began to experience full bodily support for hard and extended stress.[15]

The essential lipids had proven themselves in enabling the body to endure stress and recover from it. This makes sense, because the primary stress-coping organ of the body, the adrenal gland, is covered with lipids in an unstressed condition. These are used rapidly under

THREE VERSUS FOUR FACTOR SUPPLEMENTATION STUDY OF UNIVERSITY FOOTBALL PLAYERS

Hormone	Significance	Initial Measurement	10 Weeks Later With 3 Factor Supplement	10 Weeks Later With 4 Factor Supplement
Pituitary "The Master Gland"	Anterior pituitary hormones direct and mobilize both catabolic (tearing down) and anabolic (building up) process in the body. This gland controls breakdown of protein for fuel and building of replacement protein.	Normal: 35.0 units 23 athletes showed only 7.0 to 12.0 units 3 athletes approached	No detectable increase in pituitary output.	Every member had reached or closely approached normal output.
Estrogens "Female Sex Hormones"	High estrogen values in the male show a trend toward the slowing down of muscle formation and a stepping up of fat deposition. This abnormality is part of the reason for the tendency for middle aged men to replace muscle with fat.	Normal: 10.0 mcgm. In every case athletes showed about two times this.	No improvement had been made.	Normal reached in all but one case.
Androgens "Male Sex Hormones"	Androgens carry the steroid hormones which do much to control digestion, conversions and transportation of proteins, fats, and carbohydrates. Low levels indicate normal functions are being checked or warped handicapping the athletes.	Normal: 4.5 mgm. Athletes Athletes showed from 2.7 to 3.5 mgm.	No improvement	Rose to or close to normal.
Mineral-corticoids (from Adrenal Cortex)	Control passage of water into and out of cells by controlling minerals. Water retention or dehydration can stop vital functions and speed the aging process. They also play a part in the inflamatory response to injury.	Normal: 0.9 mgm Athletes were found to be just below to just above half of normal.	Remained in below normal	Rose into normal range.
Glucocorticoids	Enables the body to properly use glucose — the body's prime energy food. Protein was apparently being broken down for energy to supplement deficient carbohydrate conversion and oxidation.	Normal: 0.8 mgm. Significantly lowered output	No change.	All rose to normal range.
17-Ketosteroids	May aid in acid-base balance. Departure from normal indicates a derangement of the steroid hormone functions.	Normal. 10.0 mgm. Critically low, sometimes only one-half of normal.[16]	No change.	Values rose well into normal range.

intense stress. Lipids are involved in the manufacture of many hormones involved in resistance to stress.

The study of university football players which follows gives an illustration of the kinds of measurements which were made in order to evaluate the effectiveness of four factor supplementation as compared to three factor supplementation.

Those given three factor supplementation were given vitamins, minerals, and proteins. Those given four factor supplementation were given vitamins, minerals, proteins, and the essential lipids.

All the young men biochemically evaluated in this test showed a lack of steroid output. Upon being fed a complete nutritional ration they were brought into the low normal field. The time required for this was about ten weeks. The time factor is important and authorities working on other projects have extended this minimal period to three months or more.

The essential lipid sources appear to be the key factor in improving the biochemical measurements. Precursors to hormone formation from such sources as alfalfa appear to be incomplete as no gains were found when these were used on the controls.[17]

ALLERGIES: EXAMPLE OF A STRESS INDUCED DISORDER

The purpose of this discussion is not to serve as an overall evaluation of allergic problems, but to explain the role that stress can play in such problems. This is due to the role that the adrenal gland, the body's key responder to stress, plays in responding to allergies. Such an understanding can help a person to understand how to deal with an allergic problem on their own.

Allergies of all kinds are the result of invasion of the body by chemical warriors such as pollens, dusts, or foods. When these invaders attack respiratory membranes they can produce hay fever or asthma. When they attack through the digestive membranes they can produce food allergies. When they attack the skin they can produce rashes, hives or skin erruptions.

A typical attack might begin when a pollen works its way through the mouth and nose and burrows into nasal membranes. Normal mucous flow over the membranes would trap pollen, but if the vitamin A in the diet is inadequate or poorly used this line of defense will become ineffective.

If the pollen enters the nasal membrane an alarm runs along the nerves to the core of the adrenal gland (the medulla). A hormone is produced which stimulates the lungs to increase oxygen supply and the heart to increase the rate of blood flow. The shell (cortex) of the adrenal gland is also activated to send forth a host of hormones.

The hormones produced by the adrenal cortex call forth neutralizing chemicals from different body cells. These are then tailored to the invader. The hormones then direct an assault on the invaders. All this happens so fast that the ordinary person is not even aware that it is happening.

The key weapon of the body in these battles among the surface membranes are called antibodies. Antibodies are collected and carried to the problem area and discharged there by cells called lymphocytes. Antibodies cannot be formed and lymphocytes cannot be discharged of their burdens of antibodies without the aid of the hormones of the adrenal cortex.

If the adrenal gland has become semi-exhausted due to poor diet, strong emotions, or physical stress, problems develop. The essential hormones to enable the body to respond to the stress of an invader will be insufficient or out of balance. The result will be wheezing, sneezing, sniffles, rashes, hives and other miseries.

It is a mistake to overlook the role that poor diet can

play in exhausting the adrenal gland. It has been found that sugar can cause a rise of 300-400 percent in the level of corticosteroids in the blood.[19] Excess sugar consumption can therefore be very wearing on the adrenal gland.

Allergy situations are usually accompanied by tissue damage and the release of histamine in the tissues. Histamine is a chemical responsible for many of the symptoms of the allergy such as watery nasal discharge, hives and edema. This is why antihistamines are helpful in allergic conditions.[19] Vitamin C and pantothenic acid have been found to work as natural antihistamines when taken in large doses. These two nutrients are both found in very high concentrations in the adrenal gland and without a doubt aid its effective functioning.

A person with any kind of allergic problem should try to give the adrenal glands a chance to rest. The best way to do this is to avoid excess stress whether it comes from poor diet, emotions, or physical overexertion.

The best diet for giving the adrenal gland a rest is a high-protein, moderate fat, and moderate consumption of complex carbohydrates. Refined carbohydrates such as sugar and alcohol can by very detrimental. Adequate intake of protein, lipids, vitamin C and vitamin B complex will help to rejuvenate the adrenal gland, and thus enable the body to cope with stress and stress induced disorders.

LIPIDS AND THE CELL MEMBRANE

The only component of the body which could be considered more basic than the endocrine glands are the individual cells themselves.

The basic building block of the body is the cell. It is plain common sense to look at this basic building block of the body and realize that both health and disease begin here. Every organ is made of cells. The key to

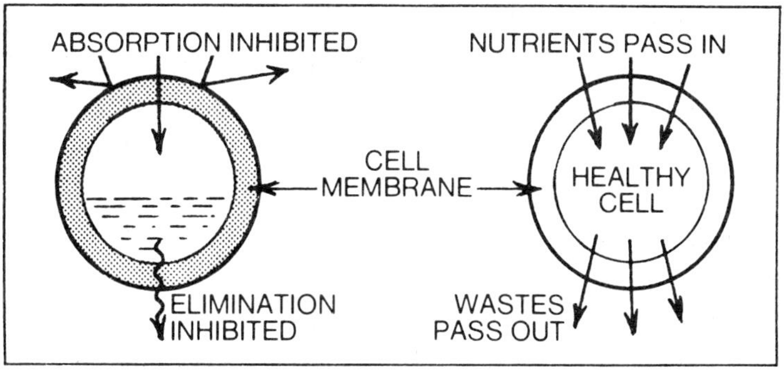

NUTRITION BEGINS WITH THE CELL

Malnutrition, particularly with regard to the high quality fats in the diet, can detrimentally affect the functioning of the cell membrane. Even though foods may be abundantly supplied in the diet they may have great difficulty in being used by the cells. The high quality fats important for construction of the membrane of the cell are known as lipids (fatty, oily or waxy substances found in fair quantities in certain seed oils such as wheat, rice and soybeans.) Modern milling and processing of foods often reduces the quantity or quality of these substances in the diet.

good nutrition begins with nourishing the cell. A disease such as cancer begins with one malfunctioning cell.

Four factor nutrition is very important for the cells of the body. Vitamins, minerals, proteins and lipids all play a role in maintaining the health of the cell. The lipids, often overlooked in nutrition, play a very important role.

The membrane of the cells of the body is composed of two layers of lipids. This bounding membrane performs at least three functions.

Firstly, the cell wall determines what shall enter the cell in the way of nutrients or other substances.

Secondly, the cell wall allows waste products and other unneeded substances to pass out of the cell.

Finally, the cell wall regulates the quantity of water in the cell.

If the body is malnourished with regard to the high quality lipids the cell wall is apparently constructed of inferior substances. The cell wall thickens and becomes impermeable. It will crumble under stress, just as bricks made of sand.

When this alteration in a cell wall takes place the basic functions of the cell are affected. Nutrients lose the ability to enter the cell. The result is that cells begin to starve and will eventually die or succumb to attack by some kind of virus or bacteria.

The elimination of waste products is also affected. Metabolic waste products and other unnecessary substances accumulate in the cell. The overall functioning of the cell will be hampered. If this happens to the billions of cells in the body it can reflect itself through a profound fatigue. We have only as much energy as the individual cells can generate.

A person moves from feeling of vibrant health to the twilight zone where they feel neither truly sick nor truly well. These people will often plague the office of a physician only to be told that there is nothing organically wrong with them. Such a health problem is often classified as being a neurosis.

The regulation of water in the cell can also be affected by malnutrition in the area of lipids. Too little water will result in dehydration of the cell, while too much will result in dropsy.

This cell wall is believed to function properly due to two different subdivisions of the lipid family.

One is an essential unsaturated fatty acid in the form of a phospholipid. This interacts with a sterol derived from the non-saponifiable (can not be made into soap) fraction of such food oils as those in cereal germs.

Both of these oils are often in short supply in the American diet due to the heating and filtering of the oils available in order to improve appearance and to prevent spoilage.

With the widespread lack of these substances both cell nutrition and cell elimination are being bottlenecked. The result is that all life processes are being slowed down and hampered. This is a threat to sustained health at all ages.

The human body is composed of so many cells that they rival the stars of heaven in number. These cells are divided into kinds such as nerve cells and smooth muscle cells. Each kind of cell serves a special function.

There are more than 1000 different kinds of cells in the liver alone. Each kind of cell requires all nutrients including the lipids.

Many cells also have a special requirement for one or more nutrients as well. For example, the thyroid cell has a special requirement for iodine. The red blood cell has a special requirement for iron. It is for this reason that the lack of one nutrient will affect one part of the body more seriously than another part.[20]

Nevertheless, all nutrients are important for health. Exclusiveness in concern about nutrition simply does not work, the body needs all nutrients to maintain health. This includes the nutrients that fall in the categories of vitamins, minerals, enzymes, protein, unrefined carbohydrates, fiber, and the lipid and sterol factors. These nutrients have been referred to as the "chain of life." This expression refers to the different nutrients necessary for the optimal functioning of life itself.

CHAPTER 6

A DIET THAT WILL SUSTAIN YOUR HEALTH

THERE is no universal diet tht will make everyone feel excellent and maintain them in perfect health. The explanation for this lies in our amazing individuality. We are all different and it is literally true that "one man's meat is another man's poison." Wheat may be a wonderful health food for one person, can create such an allergy in another that it sends him to a mental hospital.

It is also an unfortunate fact of life that our individuality makes our nutritional requirements unique. Some people are very intolerant to carbohydrates and do very well when they are restricted. Other people are very intolerant to fats, which can give them real digestive problems.

The dietary plan outlined here is therefore generalized and may have to be altered by those that have special health problems. The diet consists of basic principles of food preparation. This diet is designed to be for the healthy — and to help them maintain their health.

GENERAL PRINCIPLES

MOST FRUITS SHOULD BE EATEN RAW. Our primary reason for eating fruits is their outstanding content of vitamins A and C and their trace minerals pulled from deep in the earth by the deep roots of the trees. Vitamin C is easily destroyed by cooking, and trace minerals are often water soluble.

Fruits have often been sprayed with pesticides. It is prudent to either buy unsprayed produce or grow your own. A dwarf apple, peach or pear tree takes little space in the yard and can yield quite a harvest. Many pesticides are systemic, which means that they enter the fruit. Despite this, all sprayed fruits should be washed thoroughly and peeled. You will greatly reduce your pesticide intake.

NUTS SHOULD BE STORED IN THE SHELL. Nuts are an ideal food. They come prepackaged for long term storage. Unfortunately, when the shell is cracked nuts begin to die and spoil. Nuts which have been roasted and salted should be avoided. Roasting and salting hides the rancid taste of old nuts.

Nuts are very high in oil content. When these oils turn rancid they can be quite detrimental to a person's health. These oils are also high in calories. Eating large quantities of nuts can thus put weight on a person as easily as on the bear in the zoo that relishes them. People are much more prone to overeat roasted salted nuts than they are to overeat raw nuts. Raw nuts tend to act as an appetite suppressant. Nuts, like fruits, are an ideal source of trace nutrients because the roots of nut trees go very far into the earth searching for trace minerals.

GRAINS AND SEEDS SHOULD NOT BE REFINED. When foods are refined valuable nutrients are removed. Refining of seeds and grains usually takes place to prevent spoilage. Seeds and grains are like nuts in their high oil content. When grains or seeds are cracked spoilage starts immediately. Ideally, grains should be ground shortly before use. The whole grain should be used. Grains can often be used whole, as is illustrated by rice. Boxed cold cereals rarely have much in the way of nutritional value.

VEGETABLES SHOULD BE ONE OF THE MAINSTAYS OF THE DIET. Some varieties of vegetables can readily be grown at home in a small space. If vegetables are not fertilized with chemicals, but rather with good organic compost, they will absorb more iron, silica, and calcium, making them more resistant to insect attack. Rapidly growing greens like Swiss chard, lettuce, and spinach are ideal for home cultivation and are good for you too.

MEAT INTAKE SHOULD BE MODERATE. Most Americans eat far too much meat. Beef can have 40 percent or more of its calories in fat. That is too much fat. American farm animals often have a lot of fat on their bodies because they are raised under unnatural circumstances. Cattle are often penned up, implanted with female hormones, and grain fed to get a lot of fat on the body. The best meats to eat are those with relatively low fat content — fowl, fish, and veal. If a serving of meat does have a large fat content, eating only a small portion can be helpful.

FISH IS AN IDEAL FOOD. It is high in mineral content and contains excellent protein as well as essential unsaturated fats. Fish is a "wild" food that has not been subjected to the extensive "tampering" characteristic of so much of the American food supply. Shellfish are a risk, however, because unscrupulous fishermen will sometimes harvest them from waters contaminated with sewage and other wastes. This is unfortunate because they are exceptionally nutritious.

AMERICAN FOWL ARE RAISED UNDER GROTESQUE CONDITIONS OF OVERCROWDING. Antibiotics are often used to increase the rate of growth and to protect the consumer from salmonella poisoning once the animal has been slaughtered. Anyone allergic to antibiotics may have problems with chicken or other animals treated with antibiotics.

THE MILK DRINKER NEEDS TO EXERCISE PRUDENCE. Pasteurized milk is believed by many to contribute significantly to the risk of heart disease. Raw cow's milk can contain harmful bacteria and should be "certified" safe. Goat's milk is the closest to that of a human mother. It would be preferable to use this for formulas rather than cow's milk according to some. Cow's milk has powerful growth hormones designed to turn a calf into a cow. Goat's milk does not have these powerful growth hormones in such quantities.

CHEESES AND FERMENTED MILK PRODUCTS HAVE BEEN BENEFICIALLY SPOILED. Good quality cheese (not cheap imitation cheeses) and the better fermented milks are very nutritious and often easier to digest than milk itself. Some people allergic to milk can consume fermented milk with no problems.

GOOD QUALITY WATER IS A MUST FOR THE DIET. Water is the universal solvent which washes wastes out of the body. Many people make the mistake of only drinking coffee, tea, or cola drinks. These habits hamper the ability of the body to dump waste products.

WATER AND OTHER BEVERAGES SHOULD NOT BE CONSUMED WITH OR AFTER MEALS. Water with meals can seriously hamper digestion by diluting hydrochloric acid concentration in the stomach. It is best to drink water a half hour before a meal.

One of the best habits a person can acquire is to drink a large glass of water the first thing after rising in the morning. If the juice of a lemon is squeezed into the water it will help to cleanse the liver. Waste products accumulate in the body at night, and this will aid in cleansing the body in the earliest part of the day. The same routine at night will benefit some people.

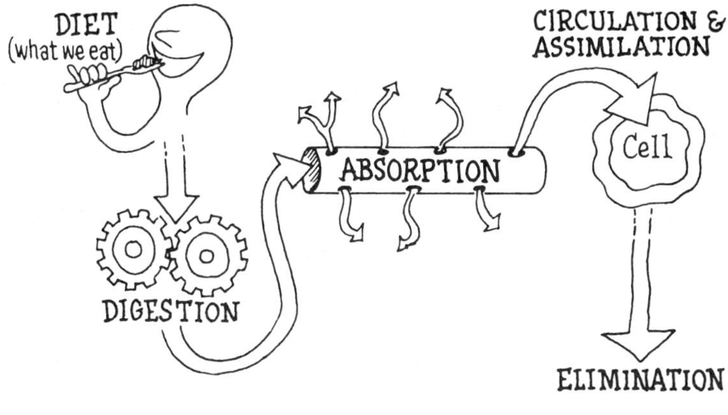

THE STAGES OF NUTRITION

1) Diet *refers to the food taken into the body. Most people assume diet is the same as nutrition, but nutrition refers to the nutrients the cells actually use.*
2) Digestion *refers to the process of breaking foods down into their component nutrients. That problems exist here is illustrated by a booming industry in antacids and digestive aids. Chewing food adequately is an important part of properly digesting carbohydrate foods.*
3) Absorption *is the process in which nutrients pass from the intestines into the blood. Many vitamin and mineral supplements are poorly absorbed because this important stage of nutrition has been disregarded in manufacture.*
4) Circulation *is the process whereby the blood carries nutrients to the cells. Good circulation can be hampered by lack of exercise and poor nutrition.*
5) Assimilation *is the process whereby the cell absorbs nutrients from the blood to use for building new cells or for repairing cellular damage.*
6) Elimination *refers to the process of removal of waste products from the body. This includes not only the part of food which can not be used by the body but also metabolic waste products, toxins, dead cells, and large numbers of bacteria from the digestive tract.*

CHAPTER 7

BOTHERED BY A BLOATED BELLY?

THE little baby boy lay in his crib. His fingers were blue, his body was cold, and he was very still. His mother looked at Philip in shock. After a few moments of frightened silence he was rushed to the hospital.

Philip's father neglected his job to be by the side of his ill son. As a consequence he lost his job. The doctors worked feverishly. They discovered that the child was suffering from a telescoping of the intestine (one part of the intestine was swallowing up another part).

The situation was critical. Philip was prepared for surgery. Doctors guessed that an infection was triggering the problem and decided to administer antibiotics to see if surgery could be avoided. With the antibiotics the problem subsided.

Unfortunately, there were subsequent attacks. The doctors watched the situation carefully, feeling that surgery might still be necessary if the problem continued. The parents began to worry. They wondered what might have created this problem.

It was at this time that they learned of my own personal experience. Upon one occasion in attempting to ward off a cold I took large amounts of vitamin C. The cold was warded off, but I developed digestive upsets. A short while later canker sores developed. I noticed a peculiar dryness in my mouth.

I went to the library and began to study viruses, digestion, *Herpes simplex* and the saliva. I learned that a beneficial bacteria called *Lactobacillus acidophilus* normally occupies the intestine. This organism manufactures B vitamins and lactic acid, a poison to many undesirable bacteria, in the intestines.

When this organism is destroyed as a result of taking antibiotics (or possibly large amounts of ascorbic acid), digestive disturbances can result. This can alter saliva flow and alter the pH of the saliva. (It is known that vitamin C is a natural diuretic and does dehydrate the body.) Change in the pH of the saliva or saliva flow can lead to cold sores, fever blisters and canker sores. When *Lactobacillus acidophilus* is destroyed, undesirable bacteria can multiply in the digestive tract creating both digestive disturbances as well as these oral complications.

When I learned this I immediately began to supplement my diet with these beneficial bacteria. The digestive disturbances and the canker sores rapidly disappeared.

As I shared this experience, Philip's mother thought back to how his problem had begun. He had been suffering from constant colds. She had taken him to a doctor for treatment. The doctor had prescribed antibiotics. A short while later the telescoping of the intestine had begun.

The boy's mother reasoned that the antibiotic the physician had given her son had destroyed some of the beneficial bacteria inhabiting the digestive tract opening the door to infection or proliferation of harmful bacteria. She began to supplement his diet with *Lactobacillus acidophilus*. The recurrent problem began to subside.

SIGNIFICANCE OF DIGESTIVE PROBLEMS

Digestive problems are known to be tied to many different disorders. This only makes sense because if a person suffers from an inability to digest his food he will not be able to nourish himself. Pronounced changes in the hydrocholoric acid production of the stomach have been found to be related to many different conditions including cancer, diabetes, acute infection, neurosis, severe anemia, arteriosclerosis, hypertension, metabolic and endocrine disorders, senile insanities, digestive upsets, chronic ulcers of the stomach and duodenum, and appendicitis , according to one prominent physician.[1]

Supplementation with another digestive aid, pancreatic enzymes, has proven helpful for a number of disorders. Disorders sometimes helped by enzymes include diabetes, schizophrenia, allergies, asthma, food eczema, hay fever, loose bowels, overweight, underweight, hives, arthritis, and ulcers.[2]

Digestive problems are quite widespread. Surveys of the acidity of the stomach have shown that 25-30 percent of those over 45 have no free or combined hydrocholoric acid. In a study of 3,000 patients more than 10 percent suffered from achlorhydria (lack of hydrochloric acid).[3]

CAUSES OF DIGESTIVE PROBLEMS

Digestive disturbances can arise from a number of causes. These include (1) malnutrition, (2) stress, (3) overeating, (4) poor food combinations, and (5) use of antacids, antibiotics or other substances that change the pH of the digestive tract or destroy the naturally occuring micro-organisms found there.

Malnutrition is a major contributor to digestive problems. The body needs vitamins, minerals, and amino acids to produce the hydrochloric acid and enzymes we need to digest our food. This is why these deficiencies tend to be self-perpetuating. With low production of digestive substances we lose the ability to process the food we eat and derive the raw materials we need to produce more digestive substances.

A lack of the following B vitamins has been found to be associated with HCL (hydrochloric acid) deficiency: B1 (thiamine), B2 (riboflavin), B6 (pyridoxine), niacin choline and folic acid.[4] Potassium and almost certainly other minerals are needed by the cells that produce HCL.[5] In addition to this protein is important.

Malnutrition can also affect the ability of the body to

produce pancreatic enzymes. Inadequate enzymes can result in poor digestion of protein. Inadequate protein intake makes it impossible to produce enzymes. All food addictions can lead to pancreatic insufficiency including addiction to alcohol or sugar. When the pancreas wears out the need for certain nutrients skyrockets, among these are B6, zinc, and magnesium.[6]

Overeating and poor food combinations can easily alter the digestive process. It is not terribly difficult for most people to eat more food than can easily be digested. This causes food to sit in the digestive tract and rot, creating a bloated, overfull feeling. It can lead to belching, burping, or intestinal gas. These problems are often simply due to the fact that we have eaten more food than the body's production of hydrochloric acid or pancreatic enzymes can handle. It is not healthy to overeat, and people live longer who don't. As people grow older HCL production decreases and ability to digest foods diminishes.[7]

Poor food combinations can also create digestive disturbances. Some foods are readily broken down in the digestive tract. Other foods digest very slowly and can not be rushed through the digestive tract. When these two kinds of foods are combined, the faster digesting food has a chance to putrify or rot while the slower digesting food is being broken down by the body. Fruits and melons digest rapidly. Meats and milk digest much more slowly. A meal that combines the two runs the risk of producing digestive upsets.

Antacids taken with meals can result in an HCL deficiency by neutralizing the body's own production of this valuable substance. Antacids can perpetuate a digestive problem or even make it worse if they are not needed. Contrary to popular belief, excess production of HCL is actually rather rare. Deficiency of HCL and also of bicarbonates is more common.

One of the rare situations where the acidity of the

stomach can be increased is by excessive sugar consumption. After two weeks of a diet high in sugar, acidity of the stomach was found to have increased 20 percent. Pepsin secretion had increased 200 percent. Pepsin is a protein digesting enzyme produced in the stomach. It is a result of this discovery that it is suspected that sugar is a major culprit in the development of chronic gastritis and perhaps also gastric and duodenal ulcer.[8]

As the pancreas wears out through poor eating habits, production of bicarbonates, pancreatic enzymes and insulin are hampered, often in that order. This can trigger terrible digestive upsets and allergic reactions to foods. Proper supplementation can be quite helpful.

The digestive tract of the human being is filled with billions of bacteria. Some of these are beneficial and aid in the breakdown of food or contribute nutritionally to the body by the production of vitamins. A good example of such an organism is *lactobacillus acidophilus.*

This organism naturally occurs in tremendous numbers in the healthy digestive tract. It manufactures B vitamins, breaks down the lactose in dairy products or the pectin and fiber in bulky foods and produces lactic acid, a potent killer of undesirable bacteria. *Lactobacillus acidophilus* is responsible for a high level of salivary acid phosphatase.[9]

When this organism is destroyed in the digestive tract due to the use of antibiotics, large amounts of ascorbic acid, or in other ways, digestive disturbances can result. Saliva flow may be decreased or its pH altered leading to cold sores, fever blisters, and canker sores. Undesirable bacteria can multiply in the digestive tract creating disturbances.

Supplementation with *lactobacillus acidophilus* can be quite valuable. There is good evidence that *lactobacillus bulgaricus,* a close relative of the organism we are discussing which is commonly found in yogurt, can not remain in the digestive tract. *Lactobacillus acidophilus* can apparently take root in the digestive tract and multiply. This is the organism that should be supplemented where digestive upsets exist.

Excessive fat in the diet can be a major contributor to digestive disturbances. Upon one occassion an individual told me that she had been suffering from digestive disturbances for years. She had seen doctors and biochemists and was taking a box of supplements. I suggested she try reducing the fat in her diet. When she did this the digestive disturbances disappeared. When she violated this principle and fried some liver in oil one evening she became sick as a dog with all her old problems.

The diet of many Americans contains as much as 45 percent fat. This is more fat than the body was designed to handle readily. Excess fat can tax the ability of the body to produce the fat digesting enzyme lipase. Protein digesting enzymes are hampered in their work if fat can not be handled adequately.[10]

In addition to this, it has been discovered that high levels of fat in the blood alter the ability of the body to handle carbohydrates. The insulin simply does not operate efficiently with too much fat in the diet. Diabetics can often have their insulin reduced when the fat content of the diet is reduced.[11]

In conclusion, there are a number of factors that can create digestive disturbances. Lack of adequate digestive substances often plays a major role. Poor eating habits can create digestive problems even if digestive juices are adequate. Finally, any alteration of the normal microorganisms of the digestive tract can affect digestion.

THE IMPORTANCE OF HCL

A lack of HCL will usually manifest itself by belching, bloating, burping and sometimes heartburn. HCL properly acidifies the stomach. The protein digesting enzyme of the stomach, pepsin, is inactive unless there is considerable HCL present. Thus deficiency of HCL can lead to protein deficiency.[12]

Inadequate HCL can also result in mineral starvation. Iron is not broken down properly and delivered to the red blood cells without HCL. Therefore deficiency in HCL can lead to anemia. Dr. Tuckey, M.D., famous researcher on HCL, maintained that his arthritic patients always had a calcium and HCL deficiency. HCL is very important for proper absorption of calcium.[13]

HCL also sterilizes the food that is eaten. This prevents putrefaction of food in the stomach or intestines by harmful bacteria. A healthy dog has almost twice the HCL in his stomach as that found in a man. As a result of this the dog can eat rotten meat. One half hour later the foul odor of the meat will be found odorless, because it has been sterilized by hydrochloric acid.[14]

Bacteria in food may not be destroyed if the stomach does not produce adequate HCL. Some bacteria are more resistant to stomach acid than others. The more resistant bacteria may survive if HCL production is decreased.

Many people return from Mexico with a particularly virulent bacteria which causes a disorder known as "tourista." This is a violent type of diarrhea accompanied by great pain. This bacteria can still be active three or four years after it is picked up. Dr. Tuckey, mentioned previously, found he could give his patients HCL tablets prior to their trips to Mexico and their resistance to "tourista" was dramatically increased.[15]

When there is a lack of HCL in the stomach one often finds a buildup of lactic acid, a foreign substance to the stomach. Dr. Tuckey found half a dozen patients with this problem who eventually died of stomach cancer.[16] HCL ordinarily filters into the blood where it serves the dual function of acting as a natural bacteriacide and as a stimulator of the activity of the white blood cells. When HCL vanishes from the circulation, other acids may enter the circulation to try to maintain the body's acid-base balance. These could include carbonic acid, diacetic acid, lactic acid, acetic acids, uric acid or fatty acids. These acids are not normal to the circulation. Such a state of affairs can open the way to a septic condition of the tissues which can lead to boils, abscesses and other degenerative conditions.[17]

Lack of HCL also slows down the emptying of the stomach. The stomach empties into the pylorus, the first section of the small intestine. Lack of HCL results in a spastic pylorus. A spastic pylorus can prevent the gall bladder and pancreas from emptying. The gall bladder dumps bile into the intestines which destroys bacteria not destroyed in the stomach and promotes the worm-like (peristaltic) motion of the intestine. Lack of bile can result in a sluggish bowel and constipation. If bile is not dumped it can accumulate in the liver and cause liver problems. If the pancreas can not empty it becomes enlarged and very tender (pancreatitis).[18] The protein digesting substances produced by the pancreas can actually function to break down the pancreas if they cannot be emptied into the small intestine.

DETECTING AN HCL DEFICIENCY

HCL deficiency can be detected by the Ewald test. A tube is swallowed and the contents of the stomach are pumped out and analyzed. It is not a very pleasant test as can be well imagined.[19] There is also a dye test which can indicate HCL deficiency.[20] Another technique is to swallow a small capsule with a miniature radio transmitter that can radio the pH of the stomach. Any of these tests would need to be conducted by a medical doctor.

There are some general indicators of an HCL deficiency. A person with this problem tends to avoid meat and eat a vegetarian diet since it digests more easily.

Gas and bloating develop an hour or two after eating. Bad breath is common in those lacking in HCL. Heartburn is also a frequent indicator of the problem.[21]

According to Dr. Philpott, a pioneer in the allergy field, the pH of the saliva can serve as a rough indicator of the need for HCL supplementation. Readings of the saliva pH can be taken with Phydrion paper. Normal saliva pH is between 6.4 and 6.8. If the saliva pH before a meal is below 6.4 the individual does not need HCL supplementation. If the pH is around 6.8 or higher it is an indication that the person may very well need to supplement with HCL.[22]

Some people simply take HCL tablets to see if it helps with bloating, belching, or burping after eating. If a person takes more HCL than he needs, this will result in a burning sensation of the stomach within an hour. Drinking two or three glasses of water will effectively dilute the HCL and help the problem. The very fact that drinking water dilutes the HCL in the stomach is reason enough for anyone with digestive problems not to drink with his meals. If a person gets heartburn from taking a certain amount of HCL, he should cut the amount in half, according to Dr. Tuckey.[23] HCL supplementation is risky for a person with an ulcer.

HCL SUPPLEMENTATION VS ANTACIDS

It is a simple fact that excess stomach acid is diluted by drinking water. Despite this fact, the sale of antacids is a multi-million dollar industry. In one compilation of major over-the-counter drugs I found 81 antacids listed and no mention of HCL. This despite the fact that the symptoms of excess and inadequate stomach acid are often quite similar. Frequent use of antacids can cause "acid rebound" where a person will need to continue to use antacids in order to obtain relief from recurring hyperacidity caused by the antacid.[24]

Make sure your HCL supplement is enteric coated. This is a process designed to make sure that the HCL does not dissolve the teeth. I will never forget hearing the tale of an older gentleman whose teeth dissolved as a result of drinking a solution of HCL for several years to remedy a digestive problem.

Dr. Tuckey, after 30 years of research on HCL came to the conclusion that the most effectively used form of the supplement is betaine hydrochloric acid with pepsin. This form meets the need of the body, while many other forms of HCL supplementation fall short.[25] With proper supplementation a deficiency can often be remedied in 2-4 months.

ENZYMES CAN HELP

As I disembarked from the plane, I though back to how the trip had begun. The young lady whom I was visiting was a good friend of a physician and his wife in California. Through them she had been introduced to nutritional supplements.

She had spent a year in a mental hospital. The physicians at the hospital had not been able to help her at all, so at the end of the year she checked herself out and flew to California to look for an answer. She had been suffering from horrible muscle tremors which disappeared when she supplemented her diet with calcium and magnesium. Other supplements were also helpful.

She was so helped that she decided to begin a food supplement business. I was there to provide some training. It did not take me long to realize that every time she ate she would begin crying or have an outburst of anger.

I asked her if she had digestive problems. She said, "I had a horrible bloating after eating when I was about five years of age." I said, "You still appear to be having digestive problems."

With this realization she began supplementing her meals with enzymes and other digestive aids. The problems began to subside dramatically. The day I left she had an omelet for breakfast and didn't have a strong reaction to it — a real first in her experience.

Later she went to an allergy unit at a hospital and found she was allergic to many foods. She worked to avoid foods and chemicals she was sensitive to.

My next stop on this same trip was in Texas. Here I visited with an old friend and his wife. She had been through a similar allergy unit. She found that the colitis problems she was suffering from had been brought on by exposure to gas heating. She had developed allergies to everything but 16 foods.

I visited them on Thanksgiving. She had eaten three of her allowable foods at one time and her head was stuffed up. I shared with her my experience in Michigan. She tried some enzymes and her head began to clear within minutes.

Food allergy is a strange phenomena. A person begins to react to the food he or she eats — food which should build health, not destroy it. There are many theories as to why the problem develops.

Some feel food allergy is tied to overeating. When a person eats too much the intestines are distended and particles of undigested food enter into the blood creating an allergic reaction. Many of those I have known with this problem eat large meals. If this is true eating smaller quantities of food and fasting should be helpful for the problem. Very frequently they are.

It is known that food allergies can be detected by having a person go on a five day fast. Subsequently, when foods are introduced the person reacts very strongly to the foods to which he is allergic. One of the unanswered questions in my mind has always been what would happen to a food allergy on a longer fast. Upon one occassion I talked with a lady who described a condition she had suffered from many years earlier which bore every resemblance to food allergy. She had gone on a 63 day fast (a very long fast!), and afterwards the problem was gone.

Food allergy can apparently be triggered by exposure to chemicals. There are many cases of people who have become allergic to foods and chemicals after exposure to pesticides or other man made substances. Obviously, the body has a mechanism for coping with substances that enter it from the external environment. If this were not so we would all be dead. The liver, thymus, pancreas, and adrenal glands must play a role here. Food allergy and chemical sensitivity can probably be created by change of these organs as a result of over-exposure to toxic substances.

Dr. Philpott, a pioneer in working with food allergy, has had dramatic results supplementing the diets of people with digestive aids, vitamins, and minerals. He feels that pancreatic enzymes are of particular benefit for this problem.

Without a doubt this is frequently so, I cannot forget the story of a beautiful young lady who told me she had suffered for years from every kind of allergy. It became so bad she had to quit her job — she was allergic to the dust in her office.

As she was getting ready to quit she decided to try some digestive aids sold by the girl who worked next to her. With very minute amounts of supplementation the problem disappeared almost completely. She was able to work again. How many millions never make the discovery that their health could be benefited by such a simple measure?

THE IMPORTANCE OF ENZYMES

Enzymes help us break down and digest our foods. There are two sources of enzymes available to a human being. The first is "exogenous" enzymes. These are enzymes which come from outside a person's body. An enzyme supplement would be an "exogenous" enzyme.

Raw foods contain large amounts of enzymes which can apparently help us handle the foods properly in the digestive process. Enzymes are fragile and easily destroyed by temperatures over 118 degrees Farenheight. Enzymes in foods are destroyed in the process of refining or they are easily destroyed when foods are cooked.[26]

The more enzymes present in the food a person eats, the easier it frequently is for his own body to break down those foods. Enzymes produced within the body are called "endogenous" enzymes.[27] The body produces three basic categories of enzymes or food digesting substances: lipases aid in digesting fats, amylases aid in digesting carbohydrate, and proteases aid in digesting protein.[28]

Recently some dramatic discoveries have been made with respect to enzymes. It has been discovered that overeating or eating the wrong kinds of foods can wear out the enzyme systems of the body. The digestive system can "steal" far more than its fair share of enzymes from other parts of the body. This can result in all kinds of problems.[29]

Enzymes have been reported to be valuable in aiding recovery from a number of different disorders. Dr. Edward Howell, M.D., and well known researcher on enzymes, reported that enzymes frequently helped patients with abdominal gas and indigestion, bronchial asthma, food asthma, food eczema, hay fever, loose bowels, overweight, underweight and hives. The pain of arthritis was lessened and improved joint movement was often noted. Enzymes are also helpful with food allergies, inhalent allergies, and allergies to different fabrics.[30]

Dr. William H. Philpott has found protein digesting enzymes very helpful for diabetes, allergies, and schizophrenia. The pancreas, which produces protein digesting enzymes, is the body's primary shock organ. It helps break down foods and chemicals the body is exposed to. This prevents these substances from entering the body in a form where they can create damage.

When the pancreas is overworked it breaks down and refuses to function in the proper manner. This is the state which exists in juvenile and adult onset diabetes as well as pancreatitis. The pancreas is hampered in bicarbonate production, enzyme production, and usually, least of all, in insulin production. Ironically, the diabetic is usually treated with insulin alone.[31]

As much as two thirds of the allergic reactions that take place in the body are due to high levels of substances called kinins in the body. Pancreatic enzymes block a rise in kinins, blocking the inflammatory allergic reactions that take place as a result of them.[32]

Poor functioning of the pancreas can play a key role in schizophrenia. Dr. Philpott took one patient classified as a catatonic schizophrenic. When she ate cheddar cheese, he found, she would develop sweating hands followed by a tension which progressed to rigid catatonia. The schizophrenia was caused by an allergic reaction to cheese. When this woman was given pancreatic enzymes and bicarbonate her body was able to cope with the cheese with only a minor sweating of the hands.[33]

Lack of pancreatic enzymes will inevitably lead to protein deficiency. Poor utilization of protein can create strong allergic reactions to automobile exhaust, while protein supplementation can often provide relief from these symptoms.[34] Without protein the body loses the ability to produce enzymes, which are built out of the protein the enzymes digest.

High blood sugar levels can also be brought on as a result of an allergic reaction to foods, due to a worn out pancreas. Dr. Philpott gave one young lady figs and watched her blood sugar rise to 300 mg. percent one hour later (a blood sugar over 170 mg. percent is in the diabetic range). When given pancreatic enzymes and bicarbonate in the proper manner, blood sugar did not rise after a meal of figs.[35]

Diabetes is often thought of as a carbohydrate disorder. Actually the situation is far more complex than that. The diabetic has a worn out pancreas with decreased ability to produce pancreatic enzymes in many instances. This results in poor use of protein. Diabetics also have problems using the fat in their diet, a well recognized fact.

Due to a disordered fat metabolism, diabetics cannot convert carotene, the precursor of vitamin A in vegetables, into vitamin A. Diabetics would do well to supplement the diet with preformed vitamin A.[36] A water solublized form of the vitamin would be ideal. Actually, the diabetic would do well to supplement with all oil soluble vitamins (A, D, E, and K). Vitamin E appears to help prevent the vascular deterioration of the diabetic that can result in gangrene, blindness as a result of retinal deterioration, and other problems.[37]

Because the diabetic cannot properly handle fat, levels of fat rise in the circulatory system. This decreases the sensitivity of insulin, making it difficult to control blood sugar levels.[38] For this reason the diabetic would probably also benefit from a supplement containing fat digesting and handling substances (a lipotropic adjunct). Any such supplement should contain the fat digesting substance lipase.

CAUSES OF ENZYME DEPLETION

The pancreas becomes worn out and begins to function inadequately most frequently due to general malnutrition or due to food addictions. In one study of several schizophrenics it was found that four of the eight essential amino acids were missing from the hair.[39] The pancreas loses the ability to function due to the malnutrition brought about by the processed foods which we eat.

As the body begins to deteriorate due to poor nutrition, allergic problems develop. People can become addicted to foods which trigger allergic reactions, wearing out the pancreas even more. Man made chemicals and particularly pesticides are potent allergy inducing substances. Many people have been sensitized to pesticides as a result of overexposure. Thereafter even small traces of pesticides can trigger an allergic attack.

Animals eating whole raw foods rarely develop allergic reactions. There is no recorded evidence of birds or wild animals living on a completely raw diet, and unexposed to pesticides, suffering from allergies. Both men and animals living on cooked foods develop all known allergies.[40]

ENZYME SUPPLEMENTATION

Enzyme supplementation is quite safe. If enzymes are taken in supplement form and they are not needed by the body to digest food they can simply be used as protein by the body. Enzyme supplementation can help to keep the pancreas from being overworked.

Pancreatic protein digesting enzymes work in an alkaline media. For this reason bicarbonate supplementation is sometimes helpful. Many antacids are bicarbonates and for this reason they make the small intestine more alkaline and enable digestive enzymes to function better. Bicarbonates should not be taken for at least a half hour after eating, otherwise they will affect the functioning of the HCL in the stomach. Many antacids contain aluminum and can be dangerous.

According to Dr. Philpott, the need for bicarbonate supplementation can be ascertained by examining the saliva after a meal. If the pH of the saliva is below 6.4 thirty minutes after a meal, this is a strong indication of a need for bicarbonate supplementation.[41]

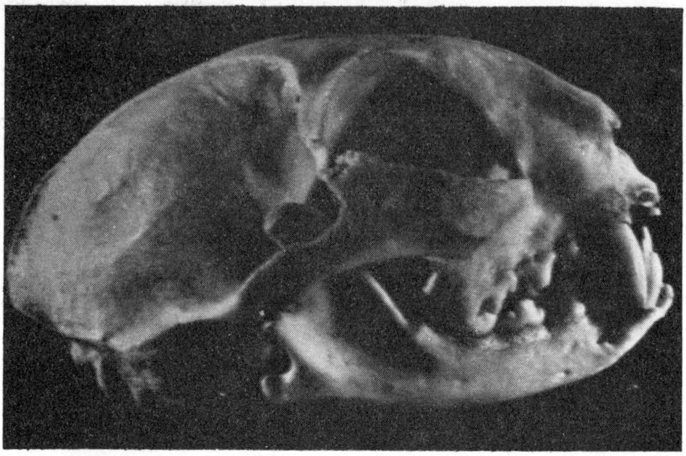

This cat was primarily a raw meat fed animal (fed cooked meat less than 6 months).

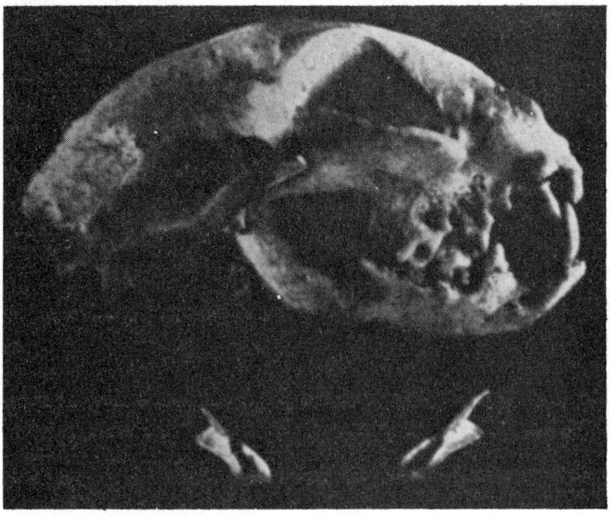

This cat was a first generation animal fed cooked meat most of her life. Note the flattening of the skull.

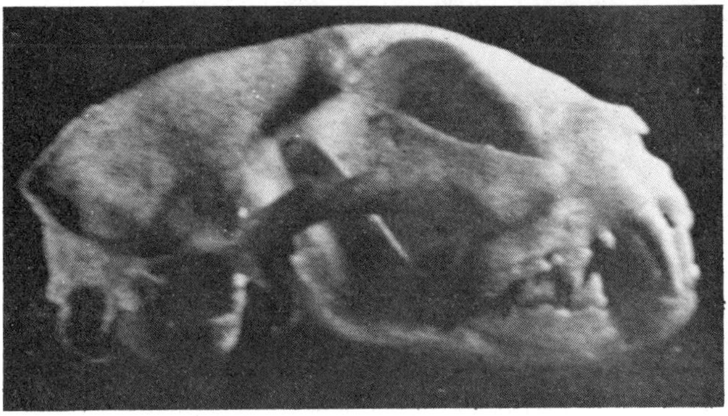

This is a male cat in the second generation of animals fed cooked meat. The flattening of the skull is obvious.

A diet of two thirds cooked meat and one third raw milk led to readily observable changes in the skulls of cats in a classic experiment conducted by Francis M. Pottenger, M.D. The structural damage that resulted from malnutrition included fine bones that could scarcely hold the skull together, small and irregular teeth, and a pronounced flattening of the skull which is readily observable in the photographs above. (From Francis M. Pottenger, Jr. "The Effect of Heat Processed Foods").

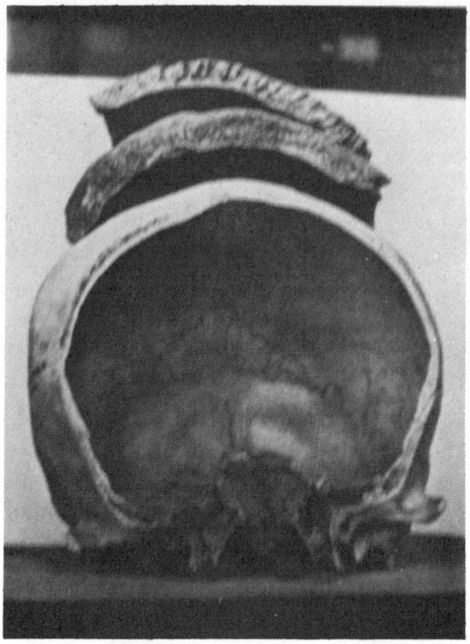

This photograph demonstrates that the skulls of the Indians who inhabited the New World prior to the arrival of Columbus were much thicker than modern skulls. These skulls came from Florida. It is fortunate that these poeple did not eat the kind of diet that we frequently do or we might not have any remains left to study. Their teeth have lasted for thousands of years and ours rarely last a lifetime. From Nutrition and Physical Degeneration *by Weston Price, D.D.S.*

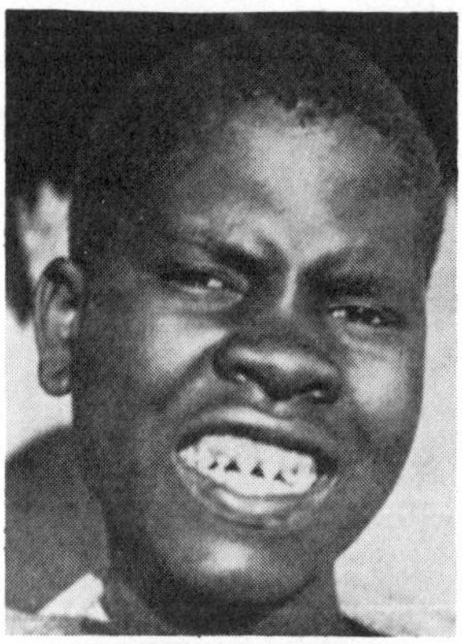

Weston Price found that the people of the Wakamba Tribe of Kenya suffered very little from dental caries even though they pointed their teeth as shown above. This was true as long as they lived on their native food. Well-nourised teeth can take a tremendous amount of abuse without suffering dental decay.
From Nutrition and Physical Degeneration by *Weston Price, D.D.S.*

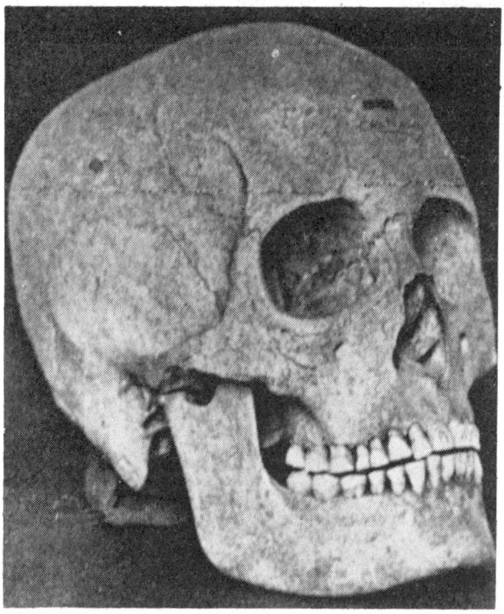

The ancient Maori of New Zealand learned their nutritional lessons well. This individual had a well formed skull with wide dental arches that provided adequate room for his teeth.
From Nutrition and Physical Degeneration *by Weston Price, D.D.S.*

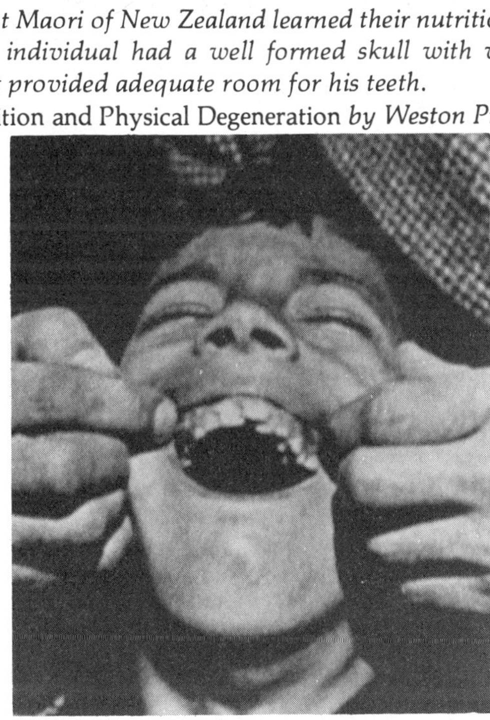

In striking contrast are the teeth and dental arches of this Maori born after the introduction of modernized foods. One of the results is narrowing of the dental arches and crowding of the teeth.
From Nutrition and Physical Degeneration *by Weston Price, D.D.S.*

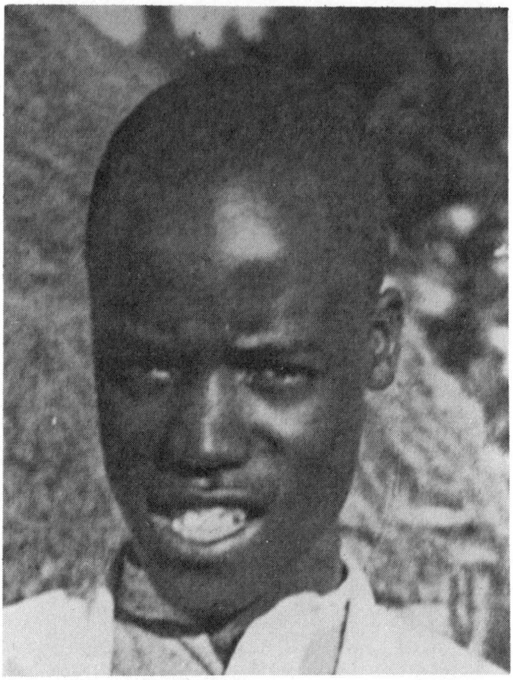

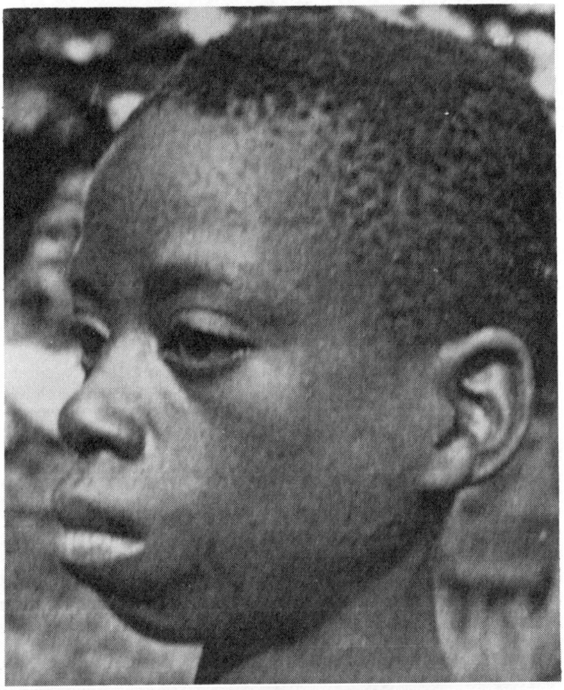

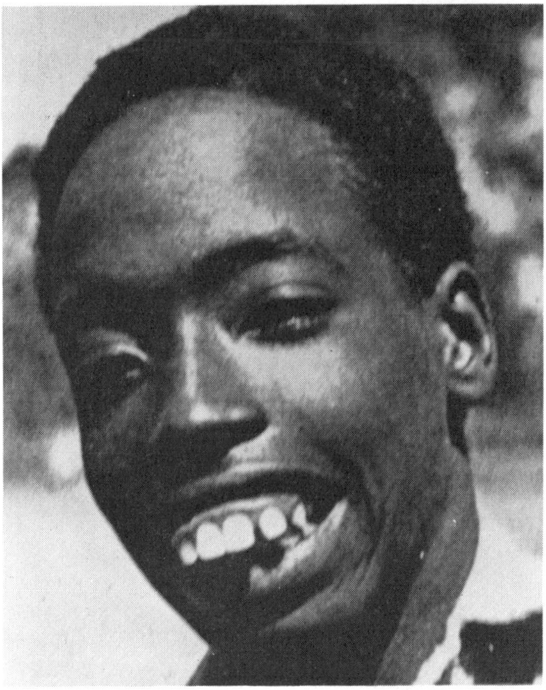

Weston Price, the great nutritional pioneer, noted patterns of physical deterioration as a result of malnutrition which extended far beyond dental caries. These changes could include such physical changes as marked narrowing and lengthening of the face (pg. 106 top), a marked depression of the middle third of the face (pg. 106 bottom), or an extreme protrusion of the upper teeth with shortening of the lower jaw (above). From Nutrition and Physical Degeneration *by Weston Price, D.D.S. Courtesy P.P.N.F.*

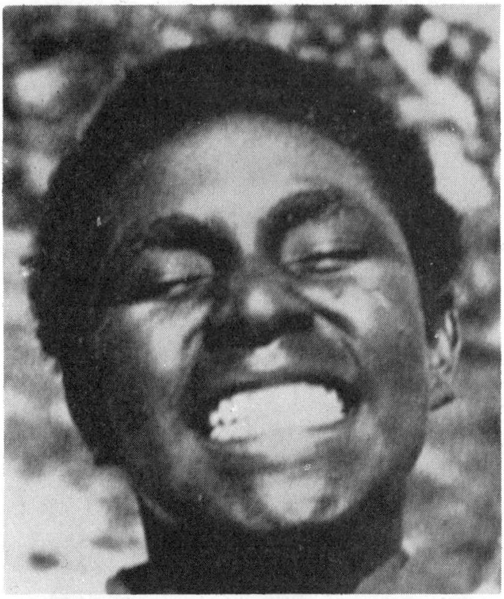

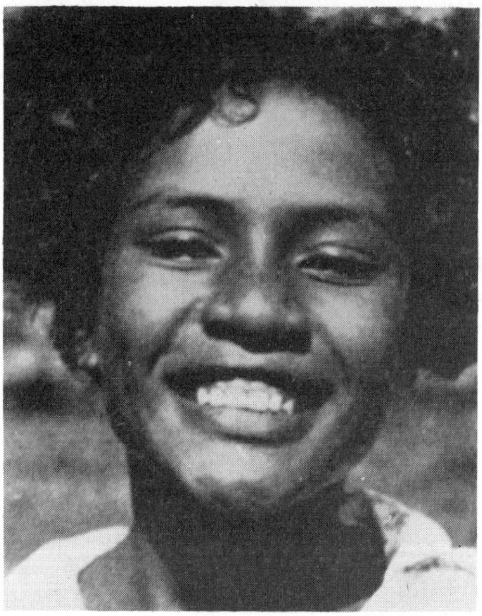

Perfect teeth resting in broad, well-formed dental arches have become a rarity. This is a testimony to the tragic nature of the decline in the quality of the American food supply. A set of healthy teeth should be the legacy of every young person, but this shall not be the case until we recognize that healthy teeth are the result of a healthy diet. From Nutrition and Physical Degeneration *by Weston Price, D.D.S.* Courtesy P.P.N.F.

CHAPTER 8

TOOTH DECAY – SCOURGE OF THE CIVILIZED WORLD

ONE of the scourges of our modern world is tooth decay. It is a problem because of its widespread nature as well as for the suffering which it causes. In 1957 one-eighth of the population of the United States had no natural teeth. Half of the population over 55 had no natural teeth. Over 98 percent of the population is afflicted with tooth decay.[1]

The tooth is like a flower or tree. Its health and integrity is to a large extent dependent upon the soil in which it is rooted. The tragedy with regard to general thinking is that we emphasize the external environment of the tooth and too frequently ignore the internal environment — the soil from which the tooth grows. Flossing and brushing of the teeth are only a minor part of what is involved in developing healthy teeth. Hundreds of civilizations have developed people with healthy teeth without paying any attention whatsoever to either of these practices.

TOOTH DECAY AND NUTRITION

Poor dental health is improved by good diet. Healthy resistant teeth can apparently throw up a wall of hardened dentin to protect the tooth when decay begins.[2] Teeth are living entities that can apparently protect themselves under the right circumstances.

Teeth are composed of minerals such as calcium and phosphorus. That these minerals can be withdrawn from the teeth has been demonstrated by studies of pregnant rats. The more pregnancies a mother rat goes through the fewer minerals are found in the teeth and the softer they become when compared to a rat that has not gone through pregnancy.[3] Most people have heard the expression "a tooth for every child." It has some basis in fact.

The lack of minerals in the diet of the average teenager may explain his great susceptibility to dental decay. He is actually in a position not much different from that of the pregnant woman. Adolescence is a period of very rapid growth, during which the body has very high requirements for calcium and other minerals to build strong, healthy bones and teeth. If inadequate calcium for example, is supplied by the diet, the teeth can have this mineral withdrawn from them to meet other bodily needs and thus become subject to dental decay.

Many young people are marginal in their calcium intake due to inadequate dietary levels of calcium or vitamin D which is necessary to properly and adequately use the mineral. Many older people suffer from a lack of calcium not only for these reasons, but also because of a declining hydrochloric acid production. This stomach acid is necessary to properly absorb calcium.

Young people can also be inadequate in calcium because of too much sugar in the diet. Sugar adversely affects calcium levels, causing the mineral to be dumped from the body. Sugar also promotes the growth of the decay producing bacteria *Streptococcus acidophilus* if teeth are not cleaned immediately after eating.[4]

For these reasons inadequate mineral intake should always be suspected in cases of "persistent" and "irreversible" dental decay. Unfortunately this information is not generally understood by the general public and even many dentists are unaware of it.

It is a mistake, however, to think that minerals are all that are necessary for healthy bones and teeth. The cells that build bones and teeth need all nutrients to function properly. For example, in one experiment children whose diets were supplemented with 3 milligrams of vitamin B6 daily experienced a 40 percent reduction in tooth decay.[5]

OUR MISDIRECTED ATTENTION

The advertising industry has done the nation a great disservice by conveying the idea that lack of fluoride is one of the major causes of tooth decay. The primary cause of tooth decay is poor diet with lack of essential vitamins and minerals and excesses of sugar and other refined foods. Despite this common sense observation government agencies for 20 years have pushed fluoridation of water supplies as a cheap and easy solution to the problem of developing healthy teeth. Small amounts of fluoride have been demonstrated to be of some benefit in prevention of dental caries, but the program which has been instituted has some basic flaws.

The campaign for fluoridation of municipal water supplies has distracted attention from the real villains responsible for tooth decay — the sugar and junk foods we consume in such large quantities that our bodies begin to fall apart. There is no real substitute for dealing with the cause of the problem. Unrelated solutions frequently just create more problems.

Fluoridation is an artificial solution to the problem of tooth decay. It cannot be successful because it does not deal with the major underlying problems. Even if tooth decay could be completely eliminated with the use of fluoridation the other harmful effects of sugar, one of the major causes of dental decay, would still impel us to avoid it. Sugar has been implicated in digestive problems, skin problems, eye problems, diabetes, ischaemic heart disease, gout, liver problems, and adrenal exhaustion.[6] Fluoride does not protect from these other harmful effects of sugar consumption.

Since fluoridation of water supplies is so frequently propounded as the final solution to dental decay it needs to be considered briefly. Two questions are immediately raised by this practice. The first is a moral question of whether it is ethical to impose fluoridation upon individuals who do not wish to have this medication in their water. The second question is whether fluoridation is unquestionably safe.

The Ethical Issue

The moral issue on which fluoridationists operate amounts to saying that some people's wishes can be ignored, because other people know what is good for them whether they want it or not. In other words it is permissible to virtually coerce patients to take drugs that many of them strongly wish not to take. The same principle that justifies adding fluoride to water would also justify adding tranquilizers, vitamins, antibiotics or contraceptives to the water. Such coercion can sometimes do more psychological damage than a mouth full of cavities.

A crucial question is not whether fluoridation will do some good, but whether the State has the right to fluoridate the water supply. The business of the medical and dental professions has customarily been to offer help to those who ask for it — not to impose treatment on those who do not wish to receive it.[7] A common sense solution to the problem would be to find a way to give people a choice of whether or not to consume fluoride.

Optimal Versus Excess Fluoridation

In 1916 mottling of the teeth was observed by a dentist in Colorado. When his observation was reported a search began for the causative agent. In 1931 fluoride was found to be the cause of the problem. It was named dental fluorosis (after fluoride).

The United States Public Health Service assigned a staff dentist, H. Trendly Dean, to determine the level of fluoride which would not cause this problem. Dean showed that this problem became detectable when fluoride concentrations rose above 0.6 ppm and at concentrations of 2 ppm or above dental fluorosis became "an acute and urgent public health problem."[8]

The dentist who had first reported mottled teeth in 1916 had noted that people with this condition had a lower incidence of dental caries than normal. Dean pursued this and found that maximum resistance to tooth decay existed at a fluoride concentration of 1 ppm. At this level only about 10 percent of the population was afflicted with mottling of the teeth. Higher concentrations only increased the severity of the mottling of the teeth and did nothing further to prevent dental decay. In 1943 the Public Health Service set this as the maximum allowable fluoridation of a water supply.

Food fluoride is as easily absorbed as is fluoride in water in most instances. Extensive investigation in the 1940's established that dietary intake of fluoride other than in water was minimal, ranging between .03 to .45 mg per day. It was later recognized that intakes above 5 mg per day can adversely affect tooth structure.

Environmental pollution with fluoride has increased dramatically since 1940. Dr. John R. Lee, MD., in a study of the unfluoridated community of Marin in 1973 found an average intake of between 0.9 to 1.5 mg. of fluoride from dietary sources.[9]

The increase in the amount of fluoride in food since 1940 is due to a number of factors. Many foods are now processed in fluoridated areas and residues are left in foods in processing. Fluoride has also become a major industrial pollutant.

The amount of fluoride emissions into the air from major sources totaled 118,700 tons in 1968. Fluorides are emitted into the air from steel and aluminum industries, combustion of coal, and the manufacture of fertilizers and other phosphorus compounds.[10]

Plants exposed to airborn fluoride concentrate the compound. Oregon state scientists found an average of 3 ppm of fluoride in 7 different crops growing in the Dallas, Oregon area. Crops were reevaluated after a new aluminum plant had been open 73 days and the same crops averaged 140 ppm.[11]

Fluorides are also being continually added to our soils. This is a result of the contamination of phosphate fertilizers with the compound. One thousand pounds of superphosphate fertilizer added to an acre will add 17.5 pounds of fluorine to the soil. The same amount of rock phosphate would add twice as much fluorine to the soil.[12]

All this rapid accumulation of fluorides in air, water, and soil is quite alarming. Reports from different corners of the globe on the toxic manifestations of excess fluoride to both plants and animals increase the seriousness of the problem.

Albert W. Burgstahler, Ph.D., reports that even 1 ppm of fluoride in drinking water can in some people result in chronic fatigue not relieved by extra sleep (thyroid depression), excessive thirst, migraine type headache, muscular weakness, sharp pains and bloating in the stomach, mouth soreness, lower urinary tract irritation, dermatitis and even visual disturbances.[13]

Dr. Albert Schatz, Ph.D., the discoverer of the antibiotic streptomycin, believes that fluoride increases the number of stillbirths.[14] Aly H. Mohamed, a professor of biology at the University of Missouri, Kansas City, has reported that as little as 1 ppm of sodium fluoride in drinking water can produce permanent genetic damage in mice. This damage is of such a kind that it could be responsible for stillbirth of offspring and thus may substantiate the observation of Dr. Schatz.[15]

Another study has demonstrated that mottling of the teeth is accentuated by malnutrition. Different investigators have suggested that vitamin A, C, calcium, and iodine are involved. There is general agreement that calcium deficiency superimposed on a diet containing fluorides has increased toxic effects and resulted in a clear reduction in the survival of laboratory animals. Fluorides administered in milk fed to rats resulted in fewer dental changes (mottling) than fluorides administered through water.[16]

These experiments suggest that perhaps a common sense means of making fluoride readily available and at the same time giving people a choice of whether or not to consume it is a possibility. Fluoridated and unfluoridated milk could be made available. This would be safer and less wasteful than fluoridating water, much of which is not consumed by human beings but simply goes down the drain.

Because the toxic effects of fluoride are worse for the malnourished, a problem is created. The battle cry of those who argue for fluoridation is that it will help the poor. This may well be true, but this is also the group most subject to malnutrition. Therefore, while fluoride runs the best chance of helping the poor, it runs the greatest risk of harming them as well.

Fluoride is a very toxic substance. It has been used to poison insects and rats and for etching glass. It is listed as a poison in the California Pharmacy Law (Article 7, Sec. 4160, Schedule "A").

Fluoride is also detrimental to plants. Soybean leaves can accumulate 200,000 times more fluoride than is in the air. This is extremely harmful to seed yield. Scientists at this time are frantically working on developing strains of soybeans resistant to fluoride, since our pollution is threatening this major food resource.[17]

Fluoride has also been implicated in the destruction of thousands of acres of forestland. This is indicated by analysis of leaves and needles for fluoride content. As animals have eaten vegetation contaminated with high fluoride levels they also have been poisoned.[18]

When it was discovered that more than a thousand acres of ponderosa pines were being damaged and dying at Lake Arrowhead, California, as a result of air pollution, a reporter for the *Herald Dispatch* did some sleuthing. He had branches taken to Griffin-Hasson Laboratories in Los Angeles. The laboratory report revealed a fluoride content of as much as 79 parts per million (enough to kill the trees). He felt a steel mill opened downwind from the forest a few years earlier was probably responsible for the damage.[19] This is the kind of damage that nothing will be done about until government agencies are willing to acknowledge that there is such a thing as fluoride toxicity and begin to do something about it.

Fluoride damage of this kind has been known for a long time. By 1893 the early German smelters had paid out 880,000 marks for current injuries and 644,000 marks for permanent relief to those who were damaged by air pollution from the smelters. For a while damage was so bad that the very existence of the smelter industry was threatened in both Germany and Britain. It was not until 1907 that it was discovered that one of the major pollutants of the Frieburg smelter was fluorine.[20]

Some people, aware of the toxic nature of some forms of fluoride, prefer to avoid it in their drinking water. We should find some reasonable way to provide them with the freedom to make that decision, through some such measure as the fluoridation of milk or alternative water supplies. The long range solution, of course, is dramatically reduced consumption of refined and processed foods.

DENTAL DECAY AND MALILLUMINATION

One final comment needs to be made with regard to our massive problem of dental decay. There is now clear evidence that malillumination (exposure to the wrong kind of light) can actually promote tooth decay. This comes as a startling discovery in the midst of an era in which we are rapidly building our schools without windows to reduce vandalism.

Immature golden hamsters fed a diet which contributes to tooth decay developed five times more dental caries when raised for 15 weeks under conventional cool-white fluorescent lighting than hamsters raised for the same period under a more innovative fluorescent lighting that approximated natural outdoor light.[21]

In another experiment twice weekly exposure to ultraviolet light reduced caries from an incidence of 28.2 percent to 15.4 percent in hamsters fed on carbohydrate controlled diets. There was an inverse relationship between hours of exposure to sunshine and the incidence of dental caries.[22]

Windowless classrooms in Sarasota, Florida supplied with full-spectrum lighting (approximating natural sunlight) reported a thirty-three and one third percent lower incidence of tooth decay when compared to a similar situation in which standard fluorescent (cool-white) lighting was used. It is postulated that body chemicals, perhaps hormones, are converted from an inactive to an active form by full spectrum light. Whether this change is initiated by effects on the skin or the eyes is not known.[23]

Full spectrum lighting is available from the following suppliers:

Solar Lighting Corporation
1520 W. Fulton Street
Chicago, Illinois 60607

Spectro-Lite Company
1621 Blue Jay Drive
Holiday, Florida 33589

Duro-Test Corporation
2321 Kennedy Boulevard
North Bergen, New Jersey 07047

SUMMARY

The widespread incidence of dental decay, narrowing of the dental arch and crowding of the teeth, nearsightedness, and other eye problems are an indicator of serious nutritional problems. We need to learn to focus on the causes of these problems (there is no one single cause in all probability). Solutions unrelated to the causes of health problems are not lasting solutions in most instances. Sometimes our patchwork solutions to health problems only serve to create more problems of a different kind, meanwhile distracting us from the underlying and unifying causes of the great majority of the health problems we experience.

CHAPTER 9

NUTRITION AND SOCIAL PROBLEMS

MANY years ago a number of nutritional investigators boldly suggested that many of the anti-social and delinquency problems our society seems to be plagued with could well be tied to malnutrition. Violent crimes of every sort have been increasing rapidly since the end of World War II. During the same period of time our diet has been deteriorating.

Sir Robert McCarrison was one of the earliest to make a comment upon nutrition and violent behavior. He reported an experiment which indicated that malnutrition created social problems among rats. McCarrison housed two groups of twenty rats each in colonies. One group was fed an excellent diet, while the other group was fed a poor diet similar to that consumed by many Englishman at that time (early 20th century).

The well nourished rats lived happily together. They gained weight and flourished. The story of the other group of rats was quite different and he reports it as follows:

> . . . their growth was stunted; they were badly proportioned; their coats were staring and lacking in gloss; they were nervous and apt to bite the attendants; they lived unhappily together and by the sixtieth day of the experiment they began to kill and eat the weaker ones amongst them. When they had disposed of three in this way I was compelled to segregate the remainder.[1]

Thus we see how murder entered rat society as a direct result of malnutrition. One wonders if a similar connection might not exist among human beings. Not only did the malnourished animals develop nasty dispositions and murder one another. But they also developed health problems including lung disease and gastrointestinal disease.

Dr. Francis Pottenger, M.D., conducted a similar experiment with cats. He fed one group of cats raw meat, while he fed another group 2/3 of their diet cooked meat. He found that cats fed cooked meat from one generation to another began to deteriorate physically.

The dispositions of the animals also began to change. He says, "Cooked-meat-fed cats were irritable. The females were dangerous to handle, occassionally viciously biting the keeper. The males were more docile, often to the point of being unaggressive. Sex interest was slack or perverted."[2] Here we see nutrition affecting not only temperament, but also sexual behavior.

What is true of animals may well be true of human beings. A London study was done of 17 delinquent girls eleven to fifteen years of age. These girls had been on a diet of white bread, margarine, cheap jam, lots of sweet tea, canned and processed meats.

When the diet was improved and diversified complexions and physical well-being improved "almost beyond recognition." The girls also became less aggressive and quarrelsome. Bad habits seemed to disappear. Problem children improved and the bored ones took a new interest in life.[3]

CHILD ABUSE AND FAMILY CONFLICTS

Nutritional deprivation can make young children behave in such a way that they are almost impossible to get along with. This can result in neglect or parental abuse.

Very young children are quite susceptible to calcium deficiency. A tiny decrease in blood calcium can lead to violent and uncontrollable temper outbursts. Babies with this problem have been known to hold their breath until they turned blue. Life with a toddler with a calcium deficiency can be a tempestuous affair.[4]

Calcium is only one of the many nutrients which can affect behaviour of a child and make him difficult to live with. Vitamin A deficiency can worsen respiratory allergies. A B complex deficiency can affect the nerves. Dr. Tom Spies found that if he told patients a funny story and they did not laugh they were quite often niacin deficient. One of the early signs of a niacin deficiency is the loss of the sense of humor.[5]

Nutritional deficiency can also contribute to birth defects, putting a strain on family relationships. Zinc provides an example of the problems a deficiency can create. Prenatal deficiency in rats results in abnormal aggresiveness in female offspring and reduces the learning ability of male animals.[6] Human beings can suffer from mental retardation when deficient in zinc during development.[7] Zinc is also involved in the normal maturation of the male. Deficiency can result in failure of the male child to develop sexually in a normal manner, resulting in many neuroses.[8]

NUTRITION AND CRIMINAL BEHAVIOR

Weston Price, one of the earliest pioneers in the study of nutrition, studied nutritional habits the world over. He found that in cultures with unrefined foods there was a much less frequent incidence of anti-social traits and lack of responsibility. In many primitive cultures prisons and asylums were found to be nonexistant.[9]

Price noted that deformity of the palate frequently accompanied malnutrition. He noted that deformities of the palate are also connected with mental functioning and behavior in many instances. In his book, *Nutrition and Physical Degeneration,* he notes observations he made that ". . . deformed palates are present in 19 per cent of the ordinary population, 33 per cent of the insane, 55 per cent of criminals, but in no less than 61 percent of idiots."[10]

Dr. Price was a dentist so he took particular note of changes in the teeth and jaw created by poor nutrition. He studied 189 boys in a Cleveland school for pre-delinquents. He found only 3 who did not show signs of nurtitional injury during the formative period.[11]

NUTRITION AND DRUG ADDICTION

Some of our major social problems like drug addiction and alcoholism are worsened by malnutrition. The role nutrition can take in overcoming these problems sometimes takes a surprising turn.

Drug addiction is a major fountainhead of antisocial behavior. The heroin addict commits crimes in order to support his habit. The severity of an addiction is often described in terms of how many dollars a day it takes to support the habit.

Alfred Libby and Irwin Stone have done a pilot study on coping with drug addiction nutritionally. As of March 1978 they had treated 150 addicts with gratifying results. Heroin addicts are treated by Libby and Stone as if they suffer from scurvy (vitamin C deficiency) and kwashiorkor (protein defiency) as well as broad spectrum vitamin and mineral deficiencies. This is in marked contrast to generally accepted methods of working with drug addiction.

Large scale drug addiction in the United States began with the use of morphine salts on wounded Civil War soldiers. Heroin was not introduced until 1890. By 1912 the rising crime rate and illegal sales of addictive drugs led to the establishment of legal opiate clinics to support the habits of users. In 1924 these clinics were closed as a horrible failure.

In the 1950's the Methadone Program was begun. The

idea was to give a legally addicting drug (methadone) in place of heroin (an illegal addicting drug). This more or less unsuccessful program is continuing today.

The concern in the area of drug addiction has centered on reducing the crimes committed by drug addicts. Little heed to the physical condition of the drug addict has been given. Without bringing total health back to the drug addict, any program is headed for failure.[12]

Libby and Stone found that they could take addicts off heroin without withdrawl symptoms. If an addict takes a "fix" during the program it is apparently either detoxified or handled by the body in such a way that there is no "high."

This ability of the body to withstand an assault of drugs is dependent upon an adequate dosage of vitamin C. It was found necessary to give between 25 and 85 grams of vitamin C for it to be effective. A $50.00 a day habit could need as much as 60-75 grams a day. These large doses were continued for 4-6 days and then gradually reduced to between 10-30 grams a day. Sodium ascorbate was used to try to get around some of the terrible digestive disturbances which vitamin C can create in such large doses.

This work on drug addiction and nutrition revealed that drug addicts lose their appetite for food and develop severe malnutrition. After a few days with vitamin C and protein supplementation a strong appetite returns and they start eating. Restful sleep also returns.[13]

ALCOHOLISM

A study at Loma Linda University in California indicates that the typical teen-age diet may contribute to alcoholism. It was found that rats fed a popular U.S. teenage diet with coffee and spices consumed 10 times more alcohol than rats fed an adequate diet. The diet consisted of "doughnuts and coffee for breakfast, sweet rolls and coffee for morning and afternoon breaks, a hot dog with mustard and pickle relish, soft drink, apple pie and coffee for lunch, spaghetti with meat balls, garlic bread, green beans, tossed salad, chocolate cake and coffee for dinner, plus a candy bar, cookies and coffee for a TV snack. To this they added eleven of the more common spices such as pepper and ginger."[14]

With this diet rats drank as much alcohol as if a 154 pound man were to drink a quart of 100 proof whiskey a day! When the spices were removed from the diet the alcohol consumption dropped in half. With both coffee and spices removed, the rats drank only one-fifth as much alcohol. When the teen age diet was changed to an adequate diet with no coffee and no spices alcohol consumption dropped to one-tenth of what it had been with the poor diet.

It was felt in this experiment that the poor diet with the stimulatory coffee and spices lowered physical and emotional resistance to stress and led the rats to drink as an anesthetic or solution to the problems they faced.[15] It is entirely possible that excessive nervous stimulation in the form of music, noise pollution, stimulating dietary habits, allergies, or sexual excesses can lead an individual to seek out tranquilizers or alcohol to calm an overly excited system.

A number of nutrients have been found helpful in dealing with alcoholism. The amino acid glutamine strongly protects bacteria against alcohol poisoning. It decreases alcohol consumption among rats, possibly by protecting the cells in the appetite center from being damaged by alcohol.[15] Protein supplementation in general would also probably be beneficial for the alcoholic, since it would tend to stabilize blood sugar levels.

Magnesium is frequently deficient in alcoholics. This deficiency may be partially responsible for withdrawal symptoms from alcohol and for the horrible delerium tremens.

The B complex vitamins can be very helpful in aiding the alcoholic or preventing the development of alcoholism. Some people serve a B complex tablet with each drink they serve guests in order to avoid a hangover the next morning. This simple procedure usually works.

Much more attention needs to be paid to the person suffering from alcoholism and his dietary habits. Alcohol lies at the root of innumerable social problems. Twenty percent of alcoholic mothers bear children with serious birth defects. Doctors have named this horrible deformity pattern the "fetal alcohol syndrome." At least 50 percent of all fatal traffic accidents involve a driver who has been drinking. Alcohol has resulted in innumerable broken homes, misery and sorrow, as well as lives with lost potential.[17]

The legal threshold of intoxication is a blood level of .15 percent in the United States. It has been found that as little as .025 percent alcohol in the blood can cause red blood cells to clump together. Observable vessels in the white of the eye become plugged. As these tiny capillaries are plugged up the brain is deprived of oxygen which this blood would usually carry. The brain cells die when they do not receive oxygen for 15 minutes. Once gone brain cells are destroyed forever, they can not be replaced.[18]

NUTRITION AND SEXUAL BEHAVIOR

The ultimate sex and sexual behavior of an individual depends upon the interaction of a number of factors. Genetic contribution is very important. There is also a gonadal contribution. Powerful kings of ancient times saw to it that their most trusted officials had been castrated (ex., Daniel 1:3). This not only made them safe around the royal harem, but also made them less aggressive and less of a threat to the throne.

There is an environmental or social contribution to maleness of femaleness. The way parents view and treat an offspring as well as the way the offspring views himself will influence the sex role he chooses to play. The social contribution to sexual behavior is usually fairly inconsequential when compared to the powerful role of the gonads and genes.

One of the most important contributions to sexual differentiation is hormonal. This is the contribution that is made by the male and female sex hormones secreted by the developing and mature gonad. Hormones produced by other glands can profoundly influence this.[19]

The human body is at the mercy of its hormone balance. Imbalance in male/female sex hormone production can lead to an actual physical confusion of the sexes. For example, oversecretion of male sex hormones by the adrenal gland of a female will result in masculinization of the woman. Such individuals may develop mustaches, increased growth of hair on the trunk, male type muscular development and hair pattern, voice deepening, and even masculinization of the sexual organs.[20]

Male sexual development is very closely tied to adequate nutrition. Development of the male sexual organs requires production of the hormone testosterone by the gonad of the fetus at one month of development. Secretion of testosterone does not take place again until some time between the ages of nine and seventeen. It is at this time that the secondary sex characteristics such as facial hair, muscular development, and deepening voice appear.[21]

Zinc is essential for the functioning of the male sex organs. Lack of this nutrient may be partially responsible for the observed lag of males behind females in growth. This happens to human children, but is rare in the animal world. Girls commonly mature two years before boys in the United States.[22] Without adequate zinc and vitamin B6 the male sex organs may not develop to full size and secondary sex characteristics may not appear.[23]

Zinc deficiency in the girl can result in failure to have a regularly established menstrual cycle until age fourteen to seventeen. The menses may start at thirteen only to skip months or a year.[24]

Delicate hormone balances can be upset by intake of estrogens as in the birth control pill. Prevention of pregnancy is the result of a hormonal change when a birth control pill is taken. Unfortunately, these same hormone changes can increase risk of breast and uterine cancer.[25]

John Yudkin, M.D., world renowned expert on the effects of sugar on the body, believes sugar alters hormone levels in the body resulting in early sex maturity. He feels this effect is due to the stimulatory effect of sugar on the adrenal gland. Pigs receiving sugar become sexually more active.

More studies have been done on girls than boys in this area. The explanation for this lies in the fact that the onset of maturity of a female is easily dated by the onset of menstrual periods. Each decade of the last century has seen a decrease of some 3 or 4 months in the age at which puberty begins for the female. The age at which Norwegian girls reach puberty fell from about 17 to 13 in the last 120 years, a drop of about 4 years. Since 1900 the age of puberty of American girls has fallen from 14 years 3 months to 12 years.[26] Sugar is only one illustration of the potent role diet can play in altering sexual functioning.

Alterations in lighting have been shown to alter sexual functioning and development as well. Development of male sex characteristics of young fish has been retarded by altering lighting. It is known that the entire glandular system of animals can be affected by altering light received through the eye. This is due to the fact that the pituitary gland, the master balance wheel of the glandular system, is affected by light.[27]

The ability of light to alter sexual functioning and general body chemistry is put into practice in animal husbandry. Chickens are exposed to extra hours of light because it increases egg production. Egg production is maximized with 14 to 16 hours of light. Lambs grow 21 to 66 percent faster with 16 hours of light a day. Exposing cattle to 16 hours of light a day significantly increases growth and milk production.[28]

We do not really know how we are changing ourselves by altering our lighting. We do so with tinted lenses, windows, and indoor living with fluorescent and incandescent lighting. We also expose ourselves to hours of television without end. What effect do these things have on the body? We do not yet fully know!

Many of the sexual peculiarities of our day may be partially understood in terms of the facts we have been discussing. Obsession with sex may be partially explainable by the high intake of sugar and other substances that stimulate the adrenal gland. Feminization of men or masculinization of women may be partially tied to malnutrition and deficiencies of such nutrients as zinc and vitamin B6. Dr. Francis Pottenger, M.D., an early student of nutrition, observed this possibility and pointed it out to his colleagues over a quarter century ago:

> Experimental work with animals shows a loss of secondary sexual characteristics after two or three generations on impoverished diets. Males lose their heavy masculine frame, their make-up begins to resemble the female. Females also tend to lose their distinguishing build so that both sexes approach a state of physical neutrality. The male no longer has the strength of body that normally makes him the breadwinner and dominant personality. The female no longer has the pelvic capacity required for easy child bearing. Other undesirable changes go along with these among individuals of either sex.[29]

SUMMARY

The preceeding discussion has been only a brief indicator of the possible ways in which nutrition and other environmental factors can create or ease social problems. The range of possibilities for investigation is almost endless. Malnutrition and the resulting change in disposition may be at the root of the many divorces and broken families we see today. There is a tremendous problem with discipline in the classroom. Despite recognition that teenagers have the worst diet of any segment of the population, not very much has been done to improve the diets of our young people.

We have shown that child abuse and family conflicts may very well result from bad diet. Perhaps even criminal behavior needs to be looked at from the standpoint of what role nutrition could play in reducing violent tendencies. Drug addiction and alcoholism may not only have their roots in bad diet, but also lead to malnutrition the longer a victim is tied to these addictions. Finally, the whole sexual emphasis of our day may be influenced heavily by the foods we eat or do not eat.

CHAPTER 10

IMPORTANCE OF IMPROVING THE AMERICAN DIET

PERHAPS you have heard something like the following: "All that you need to do is to eat from the major food groups every day and you will get all the nutrition your body needs."

This is the great cliche which has been floating around in nutritional and medical circles for the last generation and this is the cliche which is used to silence all opposition and with finality settle every discussion on nutrition. In the following discussion you will find some basic reasons for re-examining this frequently proclaimed maxim or cliche.

During the entire period of time that it has been stoutly maintained that we can get all the nutrition we need in our food the health of the nation has been continually deteriorating.

Colonel Leonard G. Roundtree who was both an eminent physician and also chief of the Medical Division of the Selective Service System during World War II said,

> "We are just completing the creation of the greatest fighting force the nation has ever seen. Instead of finding rugged, virile manhood, we have found a great many of what we call five D's — defects, deficiencies, disabilities, disease, and disorders, and the number has been appalling. ."[1]

Colonel Roundtree may have been appalled in 1944, but the situation has not improved since that time. General Lewis Hershey was head of the military draft in 1953. He was forced to ask that the physical requirements under which Colonel Roundtree operated for acceptance into the armed services be lowered or (in his own words)

"The nation will be out of manpower in the next two or three years." Those standards were lowered. In 1959 with these lowered standards 73 percent of the men examined for military service were rejected. The situation has not improved since 1959. Roundtree would be apoplectic over the conditions existing today.[2]

Dr. Cheraskin has estimated that up to 80 percent of the nation's population may be suffering from poor nutrition. A study at Jersey City Medical Center showed that 83 percent of patients admitted to the hospital had at least one vitamin deficiency and 68 percent had two or more deficiencies.[3]

There are several reasons why the food that you are eating may not be fully meeting your nutritional needs. Sedentary lifestyle is one factor. Another factor is soil depletion or deficiency. Consumption of nutritional antagonists is something which is rarely heard about, but it is something which we all do. Another reason why our diet may suffer is due to the processing of our food. In the following discussion each of these factors will be considered in detail.

A SEDENTARY LIFESTYLE

Tendencies to exercise are inborn to a certain extent. In one group of 19 healthy rats of the same age one travelled only 158 feet a day while another travelled an average of six miles a day.[4] Some people have more of a will to exercise than do others. Fortunately, it is also possible for a man or woman to choose to exercise. We need to be willing to make this decision because of the benefits which exercise offers us.

Exercise functions to increase nourishment in the body. Continuous exercise has a "training effect" upon the body. The total blood supply can increase by as much as 2 pints. The body extends and builds new blood vessels and capillaries to carry this blood to every part of the body. Remember the function of the blood! It carries food to the cells of the body and carries away waste products. Healthy circulation is imperative for good health. If we do not exercise many of the cells of the body experience a form of starvation because the tissues do not receive an adequate blood supply. Cells are also poisoned by their own waste products which are not effectively carried away.

Exercise also causes blood to flow through the body more rapidly. This speeds up nourishment and hurries away waste products. A person who exercises will feel better afterwards than he did before he began to exercise.

Exercise also fills the body with oxygen. This increases the rate of metabolism. The one who exercises is able to eat more calories without gaining weight. This can amount to as much as one fourth more calories! Included in these extra calories the exerciser is permitted, will be found extra vitamins, minerals, enzymes, proteins, and lipids. This enables him to better maintain good health.

It has been suggested that exercise is valuable in weight control. One of the problems that people have in a weight loss program is that they will reach a plateau and then will not be able to lose any further weight for a considerable period of time. These plateaus are of a shorter duration when a person is on an exercise program.

Control of the appetite is very sensitive to two factors: exercise and adequate nutrition. There is an appetite control mechanism in the brain which does not operate properly when a person does not exercise. As a matter of fact it is crippled by lack of exercise.

When rats which do not ordinarily have a tendency to become obese are kept in a warm room in very small cages which restrict their movement they invariably become fat. They may eventually come to weigh as much as two or three times as much as rats which are allowed to exercise by having larger cages. When rats are kept in a chilly room they get enough exercise by wiggling and shivering to prevent extreme obesity. These experimental findings should not be surprising, because it is the practical experience of farmers that geese, cattle, and hogs can be easily fattened for butchering by confining them and not allowing them to exercise.[5]

In summary, exercise is a way of nourishing the body. If we do not exercise to an adequate extent we may not be getting sufficient nutrients to the cells of the body to maintain good health because of *poor circulation.* Secondly, the body also may not be getting sufficient nutrients in the diet becuase of a *lower caloric* intake when there is no exercise. This means not only reduced calories, but also reduced vitamins and minerals in the diet. This could prove to be a major contributor to poor health. If we eat enough food to obtain necessary nutrients we eat too much for our activity level and become obese.

THE SOIL AND GOOD HEALTH

The second reason why our foods may not be meeting our needs is that the health of the soil affects our foods. Do you remember the story of Antaeus and Hercules? Antaeus was a man who challenged Hercules to a wrestling match. Hercules picked him up and tossed him to the ground time after time without harming him. The reason for this was that Antaeus derived his strength from the earth. Hercules learned this secret so he lifted Antaeus from the earth and strangled him. The health of man is linked to the soil just as the strength of Antaeus was tied to the earth. When this vital link is broken, disease and ill health are the result. Man's link with the soil is broken by consuming food grown on depleted soils.

Soils are depleted in a couple of ways. Some soils are *naturally lacking* in certain nutrients. Soils in districts of

Florida are notably deficient in iron. An analysis was made of turnip greens grown in these districts and iron content was 56 parts per million. Iron content of similar greens grown on soil treated with iron was 238 parts per million — over four times as much![6] Note this important point: that a plant does not have minerals that are not in the soil.

Soils are also depleted through *erosion by wind and water.* This is actually a major worldwide problem. It has been estimated that about one third of the original topsoil has been carried away from the agricultural land of the United States.[7] The Soil Conservation Service estimates that 60% of all American farmland lacks proper erosion control. This results in losses of more than five tons of topsoil per acre per year. Consequently, at a minimum, a billion tons of soil erodes away annually.[8]

The American prairie tells an interesting story. The native prairie vegetation in what is now Kansas consisted of buffalo grass to the west and bluestem grass to the east. No barrier separated the two. What is surprising is that the buffalo seldom entered the bluestem region, even though the bluestem grass was taller and more lush than the buffalo grass!

The buffalo were more intelligent than many people. They knew instinctively that the buffalo grass contained, and the bluestem lacked, the calcium and phosphorus required for their massive skeletons. In western Kansas there is a layer of calcium carbonate about one foot thick and about one foot from the surface. As one travels eastward this layer of calcium becomes thinner and deeper until it disappears.[9]

This land became some of the prime wheat growing land in the country. During World War II western Kansas produced wheat with about 18 percent protein content. Eastern Kansas wheat had only about 10 percent protein. Not only this, but western Kansas could produce 40 bushels of wheat per acre with 25 inches of rain, while

Missouri with 40 inches of rainfall was doing well to yield 25 bushels of wheat per acre.[10]

The quality of American wheat has declined. In 1900 good quality American wheat contained 12-24 percent protein. Today it is usually somewhere between 8-10 percent. It need not be this way. By carefully guarding and building of the soil it should be possible to produce a wheat that is 32 percent protein.[11]

A number of things have happened to produce this change in soil quality. In many areas of the country forests and grasslands have been destroyed by *lumbering and overgrazing.* There no longer remains a mulch of vegetation over the land to trap water and allow it to be absorbed into the earth. When rain falls if runs off quickly, eroding the soil. Rain water does not enter the ground and form underground pools, lakes, and rivers. The water table sinks and deserts are slowly formed. There were once great forests throughout the Middle East and North Africa where now there are only great deserts.

A second factor in the loss of the soil is *deep plowing and turning the soil.* In 1889 when Oklahoma was opened up for settlement a Cherokee Indian stood and watched one of the pioneers struggling to turn the thick sod over to plant his crops. The farmer went over to the Indian to ask what he wanted. The Indian pointed to the newly plowed ground and said, "Wrong side up." He then walked off. The farmer no doubt muttered something about those "poor barbarians" and went back to plowing the soil. Little more than a year later Congress declared Oklahoma a "disaster area" as winds carried the soil away by the ton.

In 1934, 800 million tons of topsoil were carried away from the prairie. The soil darkened the sky in the Eastern States for weeks and gusted far over the Atlantic Ocean. In 1954 (another dry windy period) over 2 billion tons of topsoil were swept away.[12]

The American Indian lived on the American prairie for hundreds of years without destroying the delicate balance of nature. Nothing blew away in dry windy years because the soil was not turned "wrong side up." Over 60 million buffalo once roamed the prairie. If something is not done to stop erosion it will one day be a desert.

A final problem in the depletion of the food supply through improper treatment of the soil involves the use of *inorganic fertilizers.* Usually these fertilizers contain the nutrients necessary for lush plant growth, but are lacking in trace minerals.

A four-year study was done in 11 midwestern states on 4,000 grain samples. Corn over a three year period declined 66 percent in copper content. There was a 25 percent decline in iron content. Calcium levels fluctuated wildly. Animals feeding in this area are becoming deficient in trace minerals and are developing stress symptoms demonstrated by convulsions, hemorrhaging, poor growth and many other diseases. We eat these grains and animals.[13] The severity of this kind of problem is forcing farmers to give attention to it more and more.

American farmers have found it necessary to use tremendous quantities of pesticides on their fields. Much of this is tied to the use of these inorganic fertilizers. The nitrogen compounds which are used result in rank growth. This rapid growth does not permit the plants to absorb a sufficient amount of such substances as silicon, iron and lime. These elements give the plant necessary firmness and power to resist insect pests. Most insects do not propagate very well on plants rich in lime and iron.[14]

What man considers pests are creatures that belong to nature's janitorial service. It is their duty to remove inferior life and dead organic material from the face of the earth and return it to the soil. The more inferior or diseased the life form becomes, the stronger is the attack by these scavengers.[15]

In summary, the soil feeds the plants that feed the

animals and us. Proper agriculture should feed and nourish the soil. Our soils are being eroded away very rapidly. Our methods of fertilizing the soil too often promote rapid but unhealthy plant growth.

When the soil is destroyed, so are the people. There are ruins of an amphitheater at the former city of Thysdrus in Tunisia which would seat 60,000 people. Today there are less than 5,000 people inhabiting the whole area.[16]

There are ruins of a Roman city called Timgad in Northern Africa. This city once had a population of 100,000. Today there are 300 inhabitants struggling to live on the eroded land. Is this happening to us?[17] Will our soil be eroded away and our civilization with it?

CONSUMPTION OF NUTRITIONAL ANTAGONISTS

A third reason why our diet may not meet our nutritional needs is the consumption of nutritional antagonists.

Sugar

There are many nutritional antagonists included in the American diet. Sugar is probably the worst of these. The body needs the B complex vitamins in order to be able to handle sugar. In nature these vitamins usually accompany raw sugar. When sugar is refined these vitamins are removed. Thus when refined sugar is ingested the body's own storehouse of B complex vitamins must be raided or "borrowed from" in order to burn the sugar for energy. This is what is meant when we talk about a nutritional antagonist. It is something which robs the body of nutrients. Sugar is a nutritional antagonist in four ways:

1. It has no nutrients.

2. It is a substitute for more nutritious foods.
3. It causes the excretion of certain nutrients, for example, sugar causes excretion of calcium.
4. It requires nutrients to metabolize it: B vitamins, zinc, chromium, and magnesium.

It is easy to see how the body can be depleted of these elements when one realizes that the "average" American consumes 120 pounds of sugar a year. Among teenage boys sugar may supply as much as 50% of the calories in the diet. An adult may have one fourth of his diet sugar.

The following are some "good" points to be aware of about sugar:

1. It provides a very good food for bacteria that cause dental decay.
2. It increases the acidity of the stomach and may contribute to ulcers.
3. People with one kind of skin *problem* were found to consume over 50% more sugar than those who did not have the problem.
4. Rats given a low protein, high sugar diet develop irreversible myopia or nearsightedness.
5. There is a positive correlation between diabetes mellitus and sugar consumption 20 years earlier, indicating that many of us have the ability to resist this factor for about 20 years.
6. Sugar increases triglyceride and cholesterol in the aortic wall of rats. It is a factor in obesity and heart problems.[19]
7. The activity of white blood cells drops significantly after drinking a single king sized cola drink. The action lasts for hours. This action was found to come from the sugar in the drink. The activity of the white blood cells enables them to combat invading bacteria in the body. This may explain why Americans so frequently need antibiotics. The irony is that drugs also slow down the activity

of the white blood cells in many instances.[20]

Alcohol

Another nutritional antagonist is alcohol. Alcohol is just sugar that has been run through the metabolism of a yeast plant. It has many of the same effects on the body, including the fact that it depletes the body of some of the B complex vitamins and zinc.

Smoking

A third nutritional antagonist is smoking. Each cigarette removes the amount of vitamin C from the body that is in one orange. This habit also releases cyanide, a deadly poison, into the lungs. The body uses vitamin B12 to neutralize this poison and render it harmless. Tobacco smoke also contains cadmium, another poison, which takes the place of zinc in the body.

Drugs

A fourth nutritional antagonist can be drugs. Drugs frequently destroy vitamins A, B, C, and E. Whether or not a vitamin is destroyed depends upon the nature of the drug and the quantities used.

Vitamin Antagonists in Foods

A fifth vitamin antagonist can be substances in food themselves. Many foods, especially seeds and grains, contain phytates which prevent the assimilation of zinc and other trace minerals into the body. When grains are sprouted the phytates are dissipated.

Some plants like rhubarb and spinach contain oxalic acid which inhibits absorption of calcium. Corn contains a substance called acetylpyridine which inactivates niacinamide. Niacin prevents pellagra. This explains why this disease was formerly so common among the poor in the South who lived largely on corn.

There are other foods which contain nutritional antagonists. For example, egg white contains an antagonist to the B vitamin biotin. Raw fish contains an antagonist to one of the B vitamins. Suffice it to say that many commonly eaten foods contain nutritional nullifiers. This is not a matter for concern if the diet is diverse and well balanced.

Food Additives

A sixth nutritional antagonist is food additives. Food additives have their effect on nutrition. In 1970 each of us consumed approximately five pounds of food additives. These substances serve many purposes. Some make foods safer, other make foods cheaper, others make food more or less nutritious. All food additives help companies make money and this is why they are used.[21]

Food additivies are the food industry equivalent of Hollywood's sex symbols. Many foods you see in the supermarket would not look or taste very good if food additives were not used. This brings us to the first observation which needs to be made about food additives. They deceive people into eating a poor quality of food because it looks and tastes good.

Some food additivies are also antagonistic to nutrients found in the body. Studies have shown that a mild riboflavin deficiency greatly enhances the abnormality-producing effect of sodium salicylate when it is administered to pregnant rats. When there is an abundant supply of riboflavin, the growing fetus is protected.[22]

Over one million young men were found seriously deficient in vitamin A according to light-adaption tests when they were drafted during World War II. Dr. Leo

Friedman, an M.I.T. biologist, discovered that an emulsifer (polyoxyethylene-(40)-sterate) caused an abnormal increase in the number of stomach cells which is often indicative of cancer, when the rats ate foods deficient in vitamin A, but not when there was adequate vitamin A in the diet.[23]

Toxic Metals

A seventh nutritional antagonist is toxic metals. The most toxic metals are lead, mercury, and cadmium. The toxic metals are very *easily* absorbed into the body, while the essential minerals are very *difficult* for the body to absorb. The toxic metals would be encountered rather infrequently in a natural environment. Unfortunately, these metals have unique properties and have many valuable industrial uses. The trend is toward increasing exposure to these substances which tend to decrease vitality and shorten lifespan.

Cadmium is considered the most toxic of these metals. It is similar to zinc and can replace it in the body. Adequate zinc intake can protect from cadmium poisoning. (Many American soils are deficient in zinc.)

Calcium is taken up over lead in the digestive tract. High calcium intake protects against lead poisoning. Low calcium intake increases lead absorption. Cow's milk, even though high in calcium, tends to increase lead absorption. Calcium should be obtained from a non-milk source.[24]

FOOD PROCESSING

The story of food processing really begins with the selection of varieties to grow. Varieties are chosen that will look good and keep well after shipment long distances. This is not always the same as choosing varieties of food that will contain the highest nutritional value.

Doctor Robert S. Harris, Professor of Biochemistry of

Nutrition at Massachusetts Institute of Technology said the following:

> "A detailed examination of data on Mexican foods revealed that in a number of instances the variety of food plant produced in Mexico or Central America was higher in nutritional value than the same food grown in the United States. The Latin American varieties were generally more nutritious. In his eagerness to produce more kernels per row, more rows per ear, and more ears per stalk, the plant breeder has sacrificed nutrient content."[25]

Major losses of nutrients occur when produce is picked green or shipped long distances. This much is evident from the taste of what is available in the marketplace.

Nutrients are very sensitive to a number of factors. Oxygen is very destructive to nutrients. Heat destroys many others, including some essential amino acids. Even light can destroy some vitamins. Water washes nutrients away.

After produce arrives at the market it is sprayed with water. This keeps it looking fresh. Unfortunately, thirteen vitamins and all the minerals are readily soluble in water. Between 20-40% of a nutrient can be lost in just a short washing or soaking. Imagine what happens when the produce is bought, taken home and cooked in water!

The process of refining foods also destroys many nutrients. A raw apple made into strained applesauce loses three fourths of its vitamin A. White rice has only a little over a third the phosphorus of brown rice. Puffed rice has only a sixth the phosphorus of brown rice.

The greatest devastation takes place when grains are processed. Wheat has between 80-90% of its vitamins and minerals removed when it is rendered into white flour. This means that all our cakes, cookies, breads, pies, pizza and crackers are being made from a depleted product. These are our basic foodstuffs!

STRESS

A fifth reason why our food may not meet our needs is stress. Any stress increases the general nutritional requirements of the body. The key responder to stress in the body is a pancake shaped gland called the adrenal gland. The vitamin C of the body is concentrated here. It should be no small wonder then that vitamin C is used up in responding to stress.

The hormones the adrenal gland produces in response to stress are composed of substances called sterols. These are a kind of fat found in whole grains. They are often lacking in the diet because of the refining process our oils and grains go through. Soybeans are an excellent source.

The B complex vitamins and proteins are also used in responding to stress. All of these nutrients should be obtained in adequate amounts by those who are under stress.

Adequate nutrition is more a qualitative than a quantitative experience. Most Americans eat enough food to fill their stomachs, but not all eat enough to satisfy the nutritional requirements of the cells of the body. It is a mistake to assume that because the stomach is full the cells are nourished.

It is actually possible to operate with a fair degree of efficiency on a marginal diet. The completely adequate diet is rather rare in nature. A single yeast cake given optimal nutrition and environment could produce a colony weighing more than a billion tons within one week. It follows from this that yeast cells are almost always denied an adequate environment and nutrition to reproduce at an optimal level.[26]

Marginal nutrition is rarely satisfactory for healthy reproduction. Farmers give their livestock the very best nutrition when they want healthy offspring. Unfortunately, human beings have not applied this principle to themselves.

It is estimated that there are 400,000 miscarriages annually in the United States. There are estimates that *one child in eight is mentally retarded.* Besides these there are large numbers of children who are malformed in other ways.[27] Robert Williams has made the following comment:

> "If all prospective human mothers could be fed as expertly as prospective animal mothers in the laboratory, most sterility, spontaneous abortions, stillbirths, and premature births would disappear; the birth of deformed and mentally retarded babies would be largely a thing of the past."[28]

It has been repeatedly demonstrated throughout the animal kingdom that a diet which will support the adult life will not be adequate to support normal reproduction.[29] Rats require about twenty times as much vitamin A for maximum reproduction as they need merely to maintain passable health and normal vision.[30]

The following excerpt from *The Globe and Mail,* a Canadian newspaper, illustrates that this principle is true of human beings as well as animals. We pay the cost every day for ignoring the importance of good nutrition for healthy reproduction.

> "A single family can perhaps most graphically paint the picture. A 29-year old mother had borne 11 children. The first eight were born without diet assistance, and all had small birth weights. One died at the age of one month. For her last three pregnancies the mother had diet assistance, and these three babies all weighed within the ideal range. A physical and mental assessment of all the children was done at Montreal Children's Hospital. The last three children were found to be normal. All of the others were found to be disadvantaged and likely to require support off and on through life.

It cost the public $125 to give the mother diet assistance, including the free milk, oranges, eggs and vitamins, for each of the normal babies. The cost to the public of maintaining a defective child throughout life in an institution or in the community is more than $100,000."[31]

Breast feeding is to be highly commended as contributing immeasurably to the health of the child. This is also, however, a stress upon the body of the nursing mother. Minerals are "borrowed" from the bones by the blood in the nursing process. It is very important that the diet supplies these minerals so that the blood can "repay" the loan. When these minerals are not in the diet, bones become excessively porous and fragile.

Lack of proper and adequate nutrition during the reproductive process may leave a mother depleted and exhausted for months or years after the experience. It may affect the child for the rest of his or her life.

The Stress of Injury and Disease

Injury and disease are stress conditions. Any kind of injury or disease increases the usage of many nutrients. Healing is speeded by an adequate intake of vitamin C, protein, and zinc.

Of special concern is mental illness. This can either be the cause or the result of tremendous stress. We know that schizophrenics burn up vitamin C at a rate ten times faster than a normal person. Vitamin B6 and zinc are frequently weak links in the nutritional chain of life for those who have this problem.

The brain is one of the most biochemically active parts of the body (along with the heart). It is these parts of the body that are most sensitive to poor nutrition and most observably suffer the consequences.

Different parts of the body tend to break down in different ways when they are poorly nourished. The heart tends to stop functioning. The brain tends to become biochemically imbalanced, which results in irrational and unusual behavior. Mental illness is often precipitated by a crisis which the body can not adequately respond to because of poor nutrition.

BIOCHEMICAL INDIVIDUALITY

There is one final reason why your diet might not be meeting your nutritional needs. We are all different and have different requirements to keep us healthy. Even Hippocrates noted that "different sorts of people have different maladies."[32] A greater than average need for a particular nutrient will tend to predispose us toward a particular disease if we do not obtain it.

Roger Williams studied sixteen sets of identical armadillos and found that they were not identical at all even though they came from the same egg! As an example, the weight of the adrenal gland varied two-fold. Adrenaline production varied as much as thirty-two fold.[33]

Examples could be multiplied. The point is that every person has unique nutritional requirements. He will feel best when those needs are met. Nutritional requirements are tremendously altered under any kind of a stress environment. The nutritional intake should be altered accordingly.

No one can determine if your diet is adequate except you. You can frequently tell by the way you feel. If you are not feeling well you might consider the moto of Roger Williams, the great American biochemist. His motto is: "When in doubt, try nutrition first."[34]

CHAPTER 11

MEDICINE IN THE 21st CENTURY

ONCE upon time a little village existed beneath a mighty dam. Behind the dam was a huge lake. As time went on the dam began to spring a leak here and a leak there.

The people of the village hired from among themselves caretakers for the dam to patch up the leaks. As time went on the leaks became more frequent and more caretakers had to be hired. Eventually the community spent all of its time caring for the dam, as leaks became more and more frequent.

The standard of living began to go down in the town. People no longer had the energy or time to plant crops for food or to weave to produce clothing, much less to produce toys for their children to play with. Soon they had to hire outsiders from neighboring villages to grow their food so that they could all work on the dam.

At the end of one spring day the dam inspector noted that all the leaks of that day had been plugged. The snow had begun to melt, putting extra stress on the dam and it had been a particularly hard day's work. As he turned his back, the whole dam collapsed at the same time, burying not only him, but the entire village of which he was a part.

Obviously, that dam should have been replaced long ago when it first began to show leaks. Unfortunately, the villagers were so close to their work, so busy patching, that they had not noted the obvious fact of the weakness of the whole dam.

When a problem is too close to us we sometimes lose the ability to cope with it. It is like the situation of the frog which can be dropped in a pan of boiling water and will immediately jump out. If he is put in a pan of cold water which is gradually heated to the boiling point, however, he will never jump out.

The preceeding illustrations show how far medicine has removed itself from truly helping people. Today we have developed a "band-aid" approach to health. When a health plan is discussed, what is really meant is a sickness plan. Health is the absence of sickness; it is a state of well-being. Our lack of concern for health may one day cause our society to come crashing down about our ears.

Fortunately, there is a little light on the horizon. Health care has changed dramatically in the last 100 years. In the future it will be far different that it is now. A number of new understandings or concepts are beginning to have an impact on the practice of medicine. Only a small number of medical men are aware of the principles which will be discussed in the following pages. An understanding of the changes taking place can be helpful in the evaluation of the medical care a person is receiving.

THE POTENTIAL DANGERS OF DRUG THERAPY

IATROGENIC DISEASE

"Iatro-genic" literally means an action that produces physicians. For almost a century, the term has been used to refer to health damage inflicted by physicians. For example, the prescription of thalidomide to pregnant women produced birth defects in many of their offspring. This is an example of health damage inflicted by the activity of physicians.

The subject of health damage as a result of commonly prescribed drugs is quite appropriate for a book on nutrition. It has recently been recognized that many drugs interfere with the use of different nutrients in the body.

Prednisone, commonly prescribed for tenderness,

swelling, or stiffness of the joints and rheumatoid arthritis not only alters hormones in the body, but also increases the requirements for vitamin B6, zinc, potassium, and vitamin C. Neosporin, a commonly prescribed anti-bacterial agent can interfere with the body's supplies of lactase, vitamin K, vitamin B12 and folic acid. Cortisone, used for allergies, arthritis and other conditions, can create deficiencies of vitamin B6, zinc, potassium, and vitamin C. It alters the metabolism of vitamin D. Even aspirin, consumed by the millions of tons every year, antagonizes vitamin B1 and vitamin C.[1]

The term iatrogenic may have arisen from the fact that the health damage done results in the need for more care by a physician. It has been estimated that "only modern malnutrition injures more people than iatrogenic disease in its various manifestations."[2]

It is, of course, unfair to lay the blame for iatrogenic disease at the door of the physician alone. Patients are often so desirous of receiving medication that the physician complies with their wishes.

Pharmaceutical companies are ever-present, encouraging the physician to use drugs. In 1973 the drug industry spent $4,500 on each practicing physician for advertising and promotion of their drugs. This is about how much a year of medical school costs.[3] Drug industry profits have consistently outranked those of all other manufacturing industries found on the Stock Exchange.[4]

It has long been known that medical drugs can be potentially dangerous. The unwanted side effects of drugs have multiplied greatly as drug potency and drug use have increased. Between 50 and 80 percent of the adult population of the United States and England take a medically prescribed chemical every 24 to 36 hours. As a result, a million people are admitted every year to hospitals because of a negative reaction to drugs.[5]

These tragic hospital admissions are the result of a number of unfortunate circumstances. Some people take the wrong drug. Others get an old or contaminated drug. Some people take dangerous combinations of drugs. Others receive injections with improperly sterilized syringes. Any of these can result in a drug induced illness.[6]

Iatrogenic disease can result from the natural side effects of a drug which is not carefully supervised, or simply as a result of a reaction to a particular drug. Lithium, for example, is a commonly prescribed drug for manic-depressive psychosis and as a tranquilizer. The level of the drug required to be effective is quite close to the level that can cause adverse side effects.

Extended use of lithium can produce thyroid gland enlargement (goiter). An overdose can produce weakness, lack of coordination, tremors or even stupor progressing to a coma. Any diuretic (urine producing substance) greatly increases the risk of lithium toxicity. In addition to these dangers, lithium can result in an allergic reaction of itching and skin rash by some people.[7] This is only one of the many drugs used by millions of Americans.

Most drugs have such potential for harmful side effects. Antibiotics can be particularly dangerous. Most people are aware of the fact that a dose of penicillin given to a person allergic to it may result in sudden death.[8] Fewer people are aware of what are called superinfections.

SUPERINFECTION

The term superinfection refers to the development of a second infection superimposed upon an initial infection under treatment with an antibiotic. Superinfections can occur because antibiotics alter the balance of bacterial populations in different parts of the body. Room for growth is given to organisms which are not killed by the antibiotic and which would not normally cause a disease because their numbers are so small in the body. When their competitors are destroyed by the antibiotic they can flourish wildly.[9]

It was always a source of amazement to me when I was younger that no sooner would I get over one infection than I would get another. Each one would very rapidly be knocked out by the appropriate antibiotic. It took me years to realize that my natural resistance to infection was actually being broken down by repeated use of antibiotics.

A superinfection is a good example of an iatrogenic (physician caused) disease. Without the initial use of the antibiotic the secondary problem would not have developed. Overuse of antibiotics can thus increase the need for the services of the physician. This is not to say that antibiotics should not be used when they are clearly needed.

I will never forget an experience with our family physician. He examined my sister and said words something like the following: "You have the bug that is going around. It usually lasts about a week. I will give you a prescription for an antibiotic in case you need it. If you take it you will not build the resistance you should and you will run the risk of a superinfection." Most people do not realize that infections will usually run their course if resistance is bolstered with good nutrition.

Antibiotics taken orally can seriously alter the normal bacteria of the digestive tract resulting in diarrhea, colitis, or other digestive problems. The addition of a living yogurt culture to the diet while taking oral antibiotics prevents the multiplication of harmful organisms in the digestive tract which creates these problems.[10]

DRUGS AND NUTRITION

At the present time a physician can be penalized for use of an "unorthodox" nutritional therapy (even if it works!), while he may escape any kind of censure for using an orthodox approach to the medical problem which cripples or maims a patient. Battles are being waged now in the areas of cancer, heart disease, and the treatment of mental illness.

One of the worst physician and health care related problems is malnutrition. One of the largest pockets of unrecognized malnutrition in America exists not in the urban slums but in big-city hospitals.[11]

One in five patients admitted to a research hospital acquires an iatrogenic disease. One in thirty of these cases is serious enough to result in death. Despite this a large pharmaceutical company has assured its readers that "iatrogenic disease is almost always of neurotic origin."[12]

The use of drugs by both physicians and patients is often short sighted. It is a common sense observation that a headache or the pain of arthritis are not the result of a lack of aspirin in the body. Many people act as if such were the case.

Taking aspirin (or some other drug) is often only a means of hiding or covering over a serious problem that should be examined, evaluated, and treated. Roger Williams, Ph.D., the famous nutritional biochemist, has said, "The fact is that medicine has become addicted to the administration of vast quantities of nonbiological medications which I should categorize as dubious or even essentially bad."[13]

THE CAUSE OF DISEASE

At the present time an evaluation of the different causes of disease is taking place. It only makes sense to try and figure out what causes a particular problem if one is to know how to deal with it. Unfortunately, at the present time many diseases have simply been classified as "of unknown origin" because no microrganism has been found responsible.

THE INFECTION THEORY OF DISEASE

The idea that microbes cause disease was first promulgated by Louis Pasteur. He met with great resistance and the medical men of his day would have none of his theory. The next generation of doctors, however, spurred on by what they could see in the microscope and by the spectacular demonstrations of Pasteur and others embraced the microbial theory of disease wholeheartedly. As a matter of fact, they probably carried the theory farther than Pasteur would have, for the common assumption came to be that all diseases were microbial in origin.[14]

This theory of disease became the foundation of modern medicine. It has led to the ability to immunize against disease like polio, smallpox and the flu. Antibiotics like streptomycin and penicillin have been added to the arsenal of medicine. Deaths from diseases like scarlet fever, whooping cough, measles, smallpox, diphtheria, tuberculosis, pneumonia and influenza have plummeted since 1850.

There is no doubt about the validity of this theory of disease. The only question is whether it is the whole picture. Microbes are undoubtedly involved in many kinds of illnesses.

The study of microbes will continue for a long time to come. It is possible, for example, that cancer is contributed to by a microbe known as Progenitor cryptocides. Dr. Virginia Livingston, M.D., well known cancer researcher, feels that this organism is definitely implicated in cancer. This organism infests polutry in the United States and is a problem widespread enough to create "nightmares" for the poultry industry.[15] This same organism is also present in schizophrenics.[16]

One of the ironies of modern medicine is that the

cause for the rapid decline in infectious diseases has been largely misunderstood. Some diseases like smallpox and tetanus were combated by immunization and others like diphtheria combated by antitoxin treatment. Other factors that came into play in reducing infectious disease in the western world are often overlooked.

Death rates from many infectious diseases began to plummet between 1860 and 1930. This was long before medicine developed effective countermeasures. Streptomycin (1947), the first effective treatment against tuberculosis, was only responsible for about 3 percent of the decline in the death rate from the disease since the early 19th Century. The story is similar for bronchitis, pneumonia, influenza, scarlet fever, whooping cough, and measles.

The real explanation for the major decrease in the incidence of these infectious diseases is thought to have been basic hygienic measures instituted in the second half of the 19th Century. These measures included purification of water, efficient sewage disposal, and improved food hygiene including the pasteurization of frequently contaminated milk.[17]

Incidence of infectious disease actually *began* to decrease even before these measures, however. Improved nutrition is probably involved here. A recent World Health Organization report on nutrition in developing countries suggests that the best vaccine against common infectious disease is an adequate diet.[18]

One of the little observed curiosities of infectious disease is the way in which one person is very susceptible and another person has a good healthy resistance to attack by microbes. One person will succumb to every virus making the rounds, while another person is rarely ill. This everyday observation suggests that there are other factors involved in the causation of disease besides the microbes themselves.

THE HEREDITARY-NUTRITIONAL THEORY OF DISEASE

Dr. Roger Williams has propounded what he calls the "genetotrophic" concept of illness. He feels that susceptibility to illness is related to two factors: "geneto" (heredity or genetics) and "trophic" (feeding or nutrition). In other words, one person may be very susceptible to illness because he has genetic requirements for nutrients which are very high, while another person may be quite resistant to illness because his hereditary requirements for nutrients are easily met by his diet.[19]

In a given illness attention needs to be given to more than just the virulence of a particular microbe. One must also examine the resistance of the individual under attack. That resistance can be built up or weakened by diet.

Without a doubt genetic inheritance plays a role in disease. Many disorders have a very large genetic component. For example, the need for insulin or thyroid tablets, lenses to correct farsightedness or nearsightedness, and even the need for dental work may be contributed to greatly as a result of a weak or faulty genetic inheritance.[20]

Inheritance determines what nutritional requirements will be and how easily they will be met. Even identical twins can apparently have widely differing nutritional requirements. Dr. Williams found that four armadillos from the same egg had variations in adrenaline production as much as thirty-two fold. This would almost certainly alter nutritional requirements.[21]

Since heredity has such an impact upon nutritional requirements, consideration should be given to two areas. The first is meeting the needs of a weakened heredity from the nutritional and biochemical point of view. The other factor is consideration of improving genetic inheritance through adequate nutrition and other measures at the time of conception and pregnancy.

This latter is what has been referred to as primary prevention — dealing with problems before they arise. In the laboratory it is possible to produce defective baby animals at will by giving mothers mediocre or poor diets. Well-formed baby animals can also be regularly produced by providing the mothers with superior diets.[22]

THE TOXEMIA THEORY OF DISEASE

This theory holds that excesses of certain substances in the body contribute to ill health. According to this theory, a septic condition of the tissues can be created by overeating, poor digestion, or by such substances as salt, coffee, sugar, alcohol, nicotine, or heavy metals. Toxemia is an inner pollution as serious as the environmental pollution of our cities.

Dr. Henry Bieler, M.D., was an early promulgator of the toxemia theory of disease. He called the toxemia theory of disease "the first cornerstone on which I build my house of health."[23] He felt toxemia originated from poorly selected food filled with artificial flavorings, preservatives, synthetics, and overprocessed ingredients. This provided too much stimulating food with too few natural vitamins and minerals from fruits and vegetables. Harmful drugs only compounded the problem.[24]

Germs seek their natural habitat of diseased tissue, rather than being the cause of diseased tissue. This is in much the same way that mosquitoes seek stagnant water rather than causing water to be stagnant.[25] Dr. Rudolph Alsleben, M.D., has likened germs to nature's janitorial service:

> Nature has a very large janitorial service whose sole duty it is to remove inferior life and dead organic material from the face of the earth. It is the scavenger corps, and includes everything from vultures to virus. The more inferior or diseased

> the life form becomes, the stronger the attack by these scavengers. This necessitates a maximum protection for our crops and animals. Insecticides, pesticides, herbicides, fungicides, bacteriacides, virucides, antibiotics, disinfectants, and an endless repertoire of death dealing poisons.[26]

What Dr. Alsleben has said about crops and animals is equally applicable to human beings. Dr. Bieler felt that the drugs used by many physicians were major factors in developing toxemia.

Practitioners of fasting frequently view toxemia as a major factor in illness. Fasting becomes a method of allowing the body to rid itself of toxic substances. Herbert M. Shelton, founder of one of the largest fasting clinics in the world clearly states the link in his mind between disease and toxemia:

> Acute so-called diseases are crises in toxemia. Before so-called chronic diseases are established many such crises develop. People should know the causes of crisis: they should know that if enervating habits are persisted in, repeated crises will evolve and that, finally, chronic disease will be established. When the function of an organ is stressed habitually by the way of life, its function becomes impaired. If the abuse is continued, organic change occurs. All organic change must be cared for early, else it reaches a stage at which it is impossible for vital redemption to take place. Those who suffer radical organic change never get well.[27]

The subject of fasting is dealt with in detail in another chapter.

There is clear evidence that excesses of foods and other substances can be fully as harmful as nutritional deficiencies. It is a well known fact that animals do not breed well when fed excesses of food.[28]

We often know what substances we are consuming that we should not be. Eating habits are learned and they are difficult to change. The following are some examples of substances that are known to be harmful:

Sugar	Excess fat	Caffeine
Cigarette Smoke	Alcohol	Many drugs
Heavy metals	Pesticides	Air Pollution
Water Pollution	Overcooked foods	

Sugar is a known villain in the discussion of dietary excesses. High sugar intake diminishes the ability of the white blood cells to operate. Table sugar is one of the best precursors to a substance called dextran, an excellent food for the bacteria that cause dental decay. Excess sugar has also been shown to contribute to excess stomach acidity, gout, heart disease and diabetes.[29]

Excess fat in the diet can also contribute to toxemia of a sort. There is no example of a people with a moderate fat and cholesterol intake who reveal any significant incidence of heart disease. Eskimos have often been quoted as an example of a high fat culture with relatively little heart disease, but a recent study has shown that they only consume about half the fat of the average American.[30]

Coffee, cola drinks, and tea can also apparently contribute to toxemia. Caffeine may be the major culprit. It has been shown to alter glucose tolerance curves which reflect the ability of the body to handle sugar. Coffee drinking increases free fatty acid levels in the blood. Caffeine also made it easier to create ventricular fibrillation in the hearts of dogs.[31]

Smoking is an obvious source of toxemia. The introduction of coal tar and other substances into the lungs can not help but produce toxic accumulations in the lung tissue. Anyone who has examined the lungs of smokers and non-smokers is aware of this difference.

Most drugs and many food additives can contribute to toxemia. They are not broken down and used as foods, but must be detoxified by the liver. Contaminants in air, food, and water can create similar problems.

Simple excesses of food can be detrimental because they interfere with adequate digestion. A digestive system that has been overwhelmed by more food than it can digest may lead to diabetes, arthritis, or other degenerative diseases.[32]

The point of this discussion is that contemporary medicine is acutely aware of the infectious aspects of disease. Awareness of hereditary and nutritional facets of illness is growing. Awareness of the contribution toxemia can make to illness is sometimes overlooked.

PREVENTIVE MEDICINE

Preventive medicine is a new medical concept. It means to deal with problems before they develop. There are two categories of preventive medicine.

Firstly, there is "primary prevention." This expression refers to attempts to improve a person's health through adequate concern for nutrition at the time of conception and pregnancy. Adequate attention to minor nutritional problems in the early years of life can prevent major problems from developing later on. Unfortunately, this form of prevention is a little too late for most of us around now, and the yet to be born child can not do anything about his nutritional state.

Primary prevention has been largely ignored, except by some concerned mothers. There are no real prospects for immense profit to motivate major American industries to study the needs of the mother and her child. Potential profit lies in letting problems develop and then "doctoring" them.

"Secondary prevention" refers to dealing with health problems of the adult before they become full blown disorders. It might involve dealing with a digestive upset before it becomes an ulcer, a high triglyceride and cholesterol level before it results in a heart attack, or an overweight problem before it becomes a case of obesity.

It is unfortunate that people are often uninterested in prevention and that our physicians are remunerated under the present system by frequent illnesses among their patients. They do not wish frequent illness upon their patients, and yet their financial survival depends on it. This has resulted in almost completely overlooking prevention and focusing on "crisis" medicine. "Crisis" medicine deals with a health problem only after it has become full blown. The medicine of the future will probably focus more on keeping us in excellent health, rather than worrying only about patching us up when we fall apart.

A NEW UNDERSTANDING OF NUTRITION

Nutrition

The study of nutrition has been more accidental than purposeful historically. Man has tended to overlook the role played by air, light, sound, and nutrients in his health. The more man has learned to alter his foodstuffs, the more he has been forced to pay attention to what he has done. The study of nutrition is the study of substances normally found in our foods that enable the cells of the body to operate properly.

The sum total of all the nutrients the cells of the body need to operate has been called the "chain of life." It is not possible for the cells to repair and reproduce themselves without these nutrients. We do not yet know all the nutrients that belong in the "chain of life", nor do we completely understand how they function in the body.[33]

Nature's Limited Nutritional Provision

Nutrition is not a "yes" or "no" proposition. A person is not either well nourished or not nourished at all. There are degrees of nourishment, although many people think they are well nourished if they eat three meals a day and do not have to see a doctor.

Signs of malnutrition may however result in symptoms which do not necessarily require the services of a physician. This might include such things as warts, muscle cramps, sensitivity to bright light, susceptibility to colds and infections, indigestion, allergies, asthma, and obesity.

A person's level of awareness and well-being can run the entire gamut from death to vibrant health. In between the two is a twilight zone where a person feels neither truly sick nor truly well.

Nature does not always provide completely adequate nutrition. This is demonstrated by the fact that a half-ounce cake of yeast will produce a billion tons of yeast in one week if given continuous good nutrition. Obviously, there are very few yeast cakes receiving continuous good nutrition.[34] The same is also true of human beings.

Two of the measures of the quality of overall nutrition of a mammal are physical stamina and intellectual capacity. The physical stamina of a rat can be increased ten fold by feeding it dessiccated liver. The maze learning ability of its offspring can be multiplied by giving the rat extra B vitamins during pregnancy. The very fact that such increases in physical stamina and intelligence can be obtained through diet clearly indicates that nature's nutritional provision is not always optimal. As a matter of fact optimal nutritional provision is probably more the exception than the rule.

Uniqueness of the Individual

One of the underlying pillars of the medicine which is coming is the idea that each person is unique and therefore has unique needs. The idea is not really new. One frequently hears the proverb, "One man's meat is another man's poison." Hippocrates, the father of medicine, said something to the effect that "Different kinds of people have different illnesses."

Even those of us that are most alike have tremendous differences. Dr. Roger Williams demonstrated this by studying identical quadruplets born to female armadillos. He found that even though they had all come from the same egg, brains, kidneys, and liver varied in weight as much as 50 percent or more. Levels of hormones and amino acids in the brain varied three-fold or more. Adrenaline content of the adrenal glands varied as much as thirty-two fold.[35]

Human beings can vary tremendously. One student had an esophagus stopped by a small grapefruit seed. On the other hand, some people have swallowed whole sets of false teeth.[36]

Our whole relationship to the world takes place through our senses. Differences here result in different world views. For example, some people are very sensitive to pain, while other are not. In one study 87 out of 97 prize fighters in New York were found to be relatively insensitive to pain.[37] This explains why some people see the world as a painful place and some do not. Compassion may be partially tied to the pain we feel when we are physically or emotionally hurt.

Physical uniqueness is dependent upon both birth and environment. Rats given a chance to experience novel situations showed an average five percent increase in the weight of the brain cortex over rats not allowed learning situations.[38]

Unique Nutritional Needs

Because people are physically unique, they often have unique nutritional needs. Size or activity of organs can influence nutritional needs. I know a person whose body temperature is always a little bit above 98.6 degrees. He must drink large quantities of water to keep from dehydrating and eat large amounts of food to fuel his system.

Nutritional requirements may vary not only due to physical factors, but also due to environmental factors. Requirements for the aged may differ markedly from requirements for pregnant mothers. The alcoholic and the drug addict may have very specialized nutritional requirements.

Supernutrition

Once upon a time I developed a little talk entitled "Secrets Your Pet Would Teach You If Only He Could Speak." The essence of that talk was that every dog knows he needs supernutrition — or at least those who package his food think so. By contrast the average American nutritionist and physician have been trained to regard mediocre nutrition as satisfactory.

Compare the list of ingredients on one of the better human cereals with a typical dog biscuit:

Popular Dog Biscuit	*Popular Cereal for People*
Wheat feed flour	Wheat Bran
Wheat Middlings	Sugar
Meat Meal	Corn Syrup
Soybean Meal	Salt
Dried Tomato Pomace	Vitamin C, B1, B2, B3, B6
Vitamin A Oil	Folic Acid
Steamed Bone Meal	Vitamin D2
Corn Meal	Zinc

Popular Dog Biscuit	*Popular Cereal for People*
Fish Meal	Iron
Dried Whole Whey	
Wheat Germ Meal	
Linseed Oil Meal	
Charcoal	
Brewer's Yeast	
Iodized Salt	
Caramel Color (Added for the buyer)	
Blood Meal	
Cheese Powder	
Iron	
Trace Mineral Mix (Potassium, Calcium, Magnesium, Copper, Manganese, Potassium Iodide)	
Artificial Color (for the buyer)	
Ginger	
B Vitamins	
Irradiated	
Dried Yeast (Vit. D)	

The question which naturally arises is, "Who is eating the better diet?" The obvious answer appears to be, "The dog!"

The average mammal lives six or seven times his maturation period. Thus a dog matures in about 2 years and lives for 12 or 14 years. A man, on the other hand, lives only about 3-3½ times his maturation period. Man matures in 20 years and lives only about 60-70 years. Part of the explanation for this difference may be that your pet is better nourished than you are.

Once after making comments similar to the above at a service club luncheon I received a call from a veterinarian. He wanted to assure me that many of the health problems he had to deal with in his animals were the result of the fact that people were feeding their pets the same food they were eating.

Dr. Robert L. Squibb, Chairman of the Poultry Department at Rutgers University once took a trip to Guatemala. He noticed that many of the children suffered from swollen abdomens, poor development, lack of energy and blackened skin with open sores.

Dr. Squibb noted that his chickens in New Jersey ate better than these children. He and a co-worker slightly altered a baby chick feed and fed it to a group of Guatemalan children. Within 3 weeks the swelling and sores were gone and 8 weeks later they were healthier than they had ever been. This experiment resulted in the development of a new, inexpensive health food called "Incaparina" in Guatemala.[39]

The idea behind supernutrition is not just to meet minimal needs of the body to prevent deficiency diseases, but to provide everything necessary for optimal functioning of the body. This can be used to prevent the development of degenerative or infectious diseases, or supernutrition can help the body and the physician to combat these ills once they have developed. At the present time nutrition is working against the physician, not for him.

The reader may be familiar with the term "Orthomolecular Medicine." This expression means working in healing with the same molecules naturally found in the body (ortho = same and molecular = molecule). It includes the use of both nutrients and also substances the body normally manufactures (such as thyroid hormone).

Sometimes the physician who practices "Orthomolecular Medicine" will also use "Megavitamin Therapy." This can be an application of the principle of supernutrition to medicine and healing.

HOMEOSTASIS OR BALANCE

The expression "homeostasis" literally means to "stay or stand in the same place." Rene Dubos said, "survival and fitness are conditioned by the ability of the organism to resist the impact of the outside world and maintain constant within narrow limits the physiochemical characteristics of its internal environment."[40]

Homeostasis is commonly referred to as the "steady state control." I will never forget sitting in a physiology class with my mind wandering. Suddenly my every nerve was jarred by a loud crashing sound at the front of the classroom. The professor had slammed a huge object against his lecture platform. He said, "You have just experienced 'steady state control.' It is the ability to cope with a change."

Sickness, aging, and ill health are marked by variations from the ordinary balance of the body. At first these departures from balance or homeostasis are small, perhaps even imperceptible, but they become greater and greater as time goes on. It may be a change in cholesterol levels, weight, or blood sugar.

We can help or hinder the attempts of the body to maintain its balance by the way we choose to live. Lack of sleep or excess sleep, for example, can unbalance the body. People tend to live the longest who sleep about seven hours a night.[41] Other factors enabling the body to maintain a balance are sunlight, avoiding excess noise, pure water, pure air, good diet, and an emotionally satisfying life.

CLINICAL ECOLOGY

A branch of medical science is arising which is known as "Clinical Ecology." It is actually rooted in the toxemia theory of disease. As man has dumped more and more chemicals into his environment they have begun to take their toll. It has been discovered that many people are chronically ill due to exposure to chemicals, metals, or foods.

Clinical Ecology tries to control the environment of a person who is ill to try to help his health problems. Many psychological and physical problems have been found to be tied to allergic reactions. Examples follow:

Swollen and stiff joints
Headache
Depression or outbursts of anger
Fatigue
Rapid pulse rate
Digestive disturbances
Dark circles under the eyes (called allergic shiners)[42]

SUMMARY

Traditional medicine made a mistake in confining itself to too narrow of a framework. Emphasis was placed upon substances which rarely occurred naturally in the body. These are called drugs. Drugs are often toxic and have resulted in a great number of physician caused (iatrogenic) illnesses.

Traditional medicine has also focused on microbes as the cause of disease. This is a valid emphasis, but it led to ignoring other factors contributing to poor health. Medicine is now beginning to take a look at other contributors to poor health such as heredity, nutrition, and toxemia. These are all involved in the disease process. By weakening resistance to microbes these factors can contribute to illness. Examination of nutrition, heredity, and toxemia can also help explain the degenerative diseases which at the present time are classified as being "of unknown origin."

A new medicine is developing with an interest in preventing diseases before they arise (preventive medicine). This is a valuable addition to our present expertise in dealing with health problems after they have become serious (crisis medicine). A new understanding of nutrition supports this new emphasis for we now realize that optimal nutritional needs are rarely met — there is always room to improve our nutrition and thus our resistance to infectious and degenerative disease.

Concern for internal and external environment will play a key part in the medicine of the future. We have dumped so many poisons into our environment and into our bodies that they are beginning to take a dreadful toll. Clinical ecology and similar disciplines will arise to deal with these problems.

CHAPTER 12

RESTORATION

THIS book began with the story of a young man named Jerry who was mentally ill. Society abandons such people because it does not know what to do with them. Fortunately, hope resides in this universe, no matter how dark the circumstances. The greater the mountains we have to climb in life the stronger we become.

The future is built upon today much more than it is upon yesterday. By our daily dietary choices we determine our own health and the health of our offspring yet to be born. Physical degeneration as a result of faulty nutrition is a fact, but so is physical and moral regeneration as a result of the right choices.

Jerry was sent to a leading mental hospital and put on massive medication which began to deteriorate his health. The doctor who was working with him insisted that his only hope was shock therapy. Otherwise the high levels of medication would destroy him.

The psychiatrist said that Jerry, due to the seriousness of his condition, had no hope of ever being normal again. He had only one chance in five of being released from his imprisonment in the mental hospital.

At this time experimental work was being conducted with nutrition and mental illness in Southern California. Schizophrenics had been greatly helped by a formula that had been developed. This formula was available to any hospital that wished to try it. The parents of the boy begged the head of the hospital to try this nutritional formula.

The physician was incensed that the parents of one of his patients would challenge his opinions. He told them that they would either consent to shock therapy or the boy would continue on massive health-destroying medication and institutionalization for life.

Jerry's parents visited him on the day the shock treatments were to begin. He said, "Mother, get me out of here, they give people shock treatments here." At that moment someone who had just been through a shock treatment and looked like a zombie walked by.

Jerry's mother walked to the side of the room and began crying. Jerry walked over, put his arm around her, and said, "Don't worry mother, everything will be all right." He did not know the suffering in store for him.

The hospital representative had said that there would be only six shock treatments, but they proceeded to extend them. After completing twelve treatments they quit from fear. Jerry was getting massive nose bleeds.

Many of the people in our mental institutions are warm hearted human beings. One of the young doctors responsible for Jerry said that he had the finest mind of anyone he had ever met. This doctor's assistant said that he had never seen anyone as loving as Jerry. He was always gentle and loving to other people, no matter what he went through himself.

Jerry's mother wrote to his German bride reporting the words of the psychiatrist to the effect that he would never be normal again. She suggested the possibility of an annulment. The girl wrote back from Germany asking that such a thing never be said to her again. She felt God had brought them together. She loved her husband beyond anything she could understand. She said she would find a way to him and take care of him.

On the occasion of Jerry's birthday his wife sent him a tape with the following words:

> Do not urge me to leave you or turn back from following you; for where you go, I will go and where you lodge, I will lodge. Your people shall be my people and your God, my God. Where

> you die, I will die, and there I will be buried. This may the Lord do to me, and worse, if anything but death parts you and me. (Ruth 1:16-17)

The young wife's friends nicknamed her "crazy" for wishing to be reunited with her husband. She was "crazy" for being willing to give up her administrative position for an unknown country, unknown relatives and with a new baby to care for.

Jerry's wife sent her belongings to the United States, but she was not allowed to enter. She lived from a suitcase, waiting for permission from the United States government to enter the country. Jerry's parents began to work to get his wife into the country. It took over a year and the help of a congressman to cut through the red tape, due to the fact that the young man was not able to sign any of the papers that would allow her to enter the country.

Jerry's daughter would be seven months old before the little family would be reunited. By the time they were reunited he would have improved dramatically.

The first step to recovery was release from the hospital. The head of a large company, at the request of Jerry's mother, wrote a letter to the young man assuring him that a job was available when he was released from the hospital. Jerry carried that letter in his pocket, close to his heart, as long as he remained in the hospital. It gave him hope for the future and a reason to keep on keeping on.

Jerry was released on a Friday, shortly after receiving the letter. He insisted on going to work the next Monday. The company was gracious eneough to permit this. As the weeks went by he improved. Unfortunately, he was unable to do his work, due to the effects of the medication on his body — he was too slow and too weak.

No one but the executives of the company knew what the problem was. The employees began to complain that he was creating a morale problem. It was decided that he would have to leave. Because of this first work experience he had the encouragement to go out and look for another job. Soon he was working again.

Upon release from the hospital Jerry began to supplement his diet with massive amounts of the B and C vitamins as well as protein and minerals. Chelated minerals restored the clarity of his mind.

A chiropracter discovered a dislocated vertebrae in the neck. It was felt that this dislocation, apparently caused by the automobile accident that had triggered the schizophrenia, contributed to the problem. This also was treated. The chiropracter developed a loving concern for the young man and refused compensation for her services.

There was also a psychological healing which took place. At a Christian conference ground Jerry met Paul. He later was to say, "By being my friend, Paul taught me the joy of living again."

A young girl at the employment agency was so impressed with the young man's courage, love and compassion, that she worked constantly to help find him jobs. She did not take any commission in order to help him be reunited with his family.

These years of sorrow ended with a special Thanksgiving celebration. Many of those who donated their help were present as the reunited family expressed their thanks. One person said she could have received no greater payment for her help than the privilege of seeing the family reunited.

Today Jerry is a productive citizen. He runs his own business. He is buying his own home and raising two children. Jerry and his wife feel that love of others and service to others is the rent we pay for the space we occupy in life — it is a thanksgiving for the ability to smile. Jerry's story is a reminder that no situation is completely hopeless to those who persevere in looking for a solution.

Nutrition is a part and parcel of this story. The study of nutrition brings one to an understanding of the rudimentary principles of life itself. When we neglect our nutrition we neglect our lives. No other activity can be successfully carried out if we neglect our nutrition. On the other hand, nutrition is not the sum total of life. It merely opens the door of our opportunity, so that man can do those things which he has the inherent potential of accomplishing when not hindered by a fogged mind and an aching body.

A FAREWELL TO FAT FOOTNOTES

1 Rensselaer, James, "Who Killed The Great Gluttons?", *Air California Magazine*, October 1979, pp. 47-48.

2 Hall, Ross Hume, *Food for Naught*, Vintage Books, 1976, p. 112.

3 Long, James, W., *The Essential Guide to Prescription Drugs: What You Need to Know for Safe Drug Use*, Harper and Row, 1977, p. 439.

4 Meynell, Paul, "For Complete Metabolism", *Your Start*, Neo-Life Company of America, p. C-75.

5 Leonard, Jon, J.L. Hofer, and N. Pritikin, *Live Longer Now*, Grosset and Dunlap, 1977, p. 56.

6 Reuben, David, *The Save Your Life Diet*, Random House, 1975, p. 103.

7 Contra Costa Times, Tuesday, October 17, 1978, p. 5.

8 Maness, Bill, "How Much Do You Know About Jogging," *Aviation Medical Bulletin*, April 1977, p. 1.

9 Leonard, Jon, *Live Longer Now*, p. 78.

10 *Ibid.*, p. 78-9.

11 *Ibid.*, p. 80.

12 Bailey, Covert, *Fit or Fat*, Houghton Mifflin Company, 1978, pp. 24-5.

13 Maness, "How Much Do You Know About Jogging?", p. 2.

14 Bailey, Covert, *Fit or Fat*, p. 36.

15 *Ibid.*, p. 27.

16 Cooper, Kenneth H., *The New Aerobics*, Bantam Books, 1972, pp. 16-17.

17 Leonard, Jon, *Live Longer Now*, p. 81.

18 Bailey, Covert, *Fit or Fat*, pp. 94-5.

19 *Ibid*,. p. 26. (Maximum Pulse - Resting Pulse x 65% + Resting Pulse = Training heart rate of 80% of maximum.)

20 *Ibid.*, p. 8.

21 *Ibid.*, p. 7.

22 Maness, Bill, How Much Do You Know About Jogging?", p.2.

23 Williams, Roger, *Nutrition Against Disease*, Bantam Books, 1973, p. 104.

24 *Ibid.*, p. 106.

25 Newbold, H. L., *Dr. Newbold's Revolutionary New Discoveries About Weight Loss*, Rawson Associates Publishers, Inc., 1977, p. 34.

26 *Ibid.*, p. 35.

27 *Your Start*, Neo-Life Company of America, 1978, p. C-51.

28 Bailey, Herbert, *Vitamin E, Your Key to a Healthy Heart*, Arc Books, Inc., 1969, pp. 9-11.
29 Cheraskin, E., W. M. Ringsdorf, Jr., and Arline Brecher, *Psycho-Dietetics*, Bantam Books, 1976, p. 142.
30 Ershoff, B. H., *Proceedings of the Society for Experimental Biology and Medicine*, vol. 77, pp. 488-491 (1957).
31 Hall, Ross Hume, *Food for Naught*, p. 112.

FASTING: LEARNING NOT TO EAT

1 Copeland, Lewis and Faye, ed., *10,000 Jokes, Toasts and Stories*, Doubleday and Co., Inc., c. 1965, p. 65.
2 Shelton, Herbert M., *Fasting and Sunbathing*, Shetlon's Health School, 1963, p. 88.
3 *Ibid.*, pp. 36-7
4 Shelton, H.M., *Fasting for Renewal of Life*, Natural Hygiene Press, 1974, p. 69.
5 Wallis, Arthur, *God's Chosen Fast*, Christian Literature Crusade, 1971, p. 82.
6 Bragg, Paul, *The Miracle of Fasting*, Health Science, 1971, pg. 10.
7 Clark, Linda, *Secrets of Health and Beauty*, Pyramid, 1975, p. 33.
8 Shelton, Herbert M., *Fasting Can Save Your Life*, Natural Hygiene Press, 1967, pp. 80-81.
9 Shelton, *Fasting and Sunbathing*, p. 218.
10 Shelton, *Fasting Can Save Your Life, p. 83.*
11 Shelton, *Fasting and Sunbathing*, p. 217.
12 *Ibid.*, p. 237.
13 Winter, Ruth, "How Fast Are You Aging?", *Reader's Digest*, November 1968, p. 161.
14 Reuters, "Unlocking Longevity's Secrets," *Reader's Digest*, September, 1971, p. 24.
15 Rodale, J. I., *The Prevention Method for Better Health*, Rodale Books Inc., 1969, p. 880.
16 Airola, Paavo, *Health Secrets from Europe*, Arco Publishing Company, c. 1970, p. 34.
17 Shelton, *Fasting and Sunbathing*, p. 217.
18 "Dieting," *Time*, January 24, 1964, p. 31.
19 Scrimshaw, Nevin S., and Young, Vernon R., "The Physiology of Starvation," *Scientific American*, October, 1971, p. 15.
20 May, Marsha, "Ted Mack: I Turned Down Elvis Presley and Tiny Tim for My 'Original Amateur Hour'", *National Enquirer*, October 14, 1975, p. 47.

21 Scrimshaw, "The Physiology of Starvation," p. 16.
22 Shelton, *Fasting Can Save Your Life*, p. 83.
23 Shelton, *Fasting for Renewal of Life*, p. 161.

THE SYNERGISTIC EFFECT AND THE CHAIN OF LIFE

1 Myron S. Lewis, "RDA", Lewis Laboratories, LTD., Westport, Conn., p. 1.
2 *Ibid, loc. cit.*
3 Linda Clark, *Secrets of Health and Beauty*, New York; Pyramid Books, 1975, p. 46.
4 Linus Pauling, *Vitamin C and the Common Cold*, San Francisco: W.H. Freedman and Co., p. 37.
5 Carl C. Pfeiffer, *Mental and Elemental Nutrients*, New Cannan, Conn.: Keats Publishing, Inc., p. 231.
6 Roger Williams, *Nutrition Against Disease*, New York: Pitman Publishing Corporation, 1971, p. 47.
7 Francis Moore Lappe, *Diet for a Small Planet*, New York: Ballantine Books, 1975, pp. 66-63.
8 Joseph S. Fruton, "Proteins", *Scientific American Reader*, New York: Simon and Schuster, 1953, p. 239.
9 Francis M. Pottenger, "The Effect of Heat Processed Foods and Metabolized Vitamin D Milk on the Dentofacial Structures of Experimental Animals", *American Journal of Orthodontics and Oral Surgery*, Vo. 32, No. 8, August 1946, pp. 467-485.
10 John Yudkin, "Sugar and Disease", *Nature*, Vol. 239, September 22, 1972, p. 198.
11 Alsoph Corwin, "Civilization and Health", *Price Pottenger Nutrition Foundation Membership Bulletin*, La Mesa, California, Vol. 4, No. 3, p. 5.
12 John Meyers and Karl Schutte, *Metabolic Aspects of Health*, Kentfield, California: Discovery Press, 1979, p. 284.
13 Weston Price, *Nutrition and Physical Degeneration*, Santa Monica, California: Price Pottenger Nutrition Foundation, 1975, pp. 142, 150, 153.
14 David Reuben, *The Save Your Life Diet*, New York: Random House, 1975, p. 29.

FOUR FACTOR NUTRITION

1 Mcquade, Walter and Ann Aikman, *Stress*, Bantam Books, 1975,

pp. 12-14.
[2] Dunnington Lewis L., *Keys to Richer Living,* MacMillan Company c. 1952, p. 95.
[3] Gibson, John E., "Strange Things 'Stress' Does to You," *Family Weekly,* March 30, 1975, p. 17.
[4] McMillen, S.I., *None of These Diseases,* Fleming H. Revell Company, c. 1963, p. 81.
[5] Dunnington, p. 76.
[6] McMillen, p. 71.
[7] Selye, Hans, "Stress Without Distress and Stress in Health and Disease," Xedia Programs, P.O. Box 20, Sunset Beach, California, 90742.
[8] Selye, Hans, *The Stress of Life,* McGraw Hill, c. 1956, pp. 15-18.
[9] Constantinides, P.C. and Niall Carey, "The Alarm Reaction," *Scientific American Reader,* Simon and Schuster, 1953, pp. 395-399.
[10] Gray, George W., "ACTH and Cortisone," *Scientific American Reader,* Simon and Schuster, 1953, p. 382.
[11] *Ibid.,* p. 382-3.
[12] *Ibid.,* p. 385.
[13] *Ibid.,* p. 387.
[14] Meynell, Paul, "Health: Chemical Balance", *Your Start,* Neo-Life Company of America, 1978, p. C-73-4.
[15] Meynell, Paul, "For Improved Metabolism," *Your Start,* Neo-LIfe Company of America, 1978, p. C-77-8.
[16] Meynell, Paul, "For Complete Metabolism," *Your Start,* Neo-Life Company of America, 1978, p. C-75-6.
[17] *Ibid., loc. cit.*
[18] Yudkin, John, "Sugar and Disease," *Nature,* September 22, 1972, p. 199.
[19] McClintic, J. Robert, *Physiology of the Human Body,* John Wiley and Sons, Inc., c. 1975, p. 121.
[20] Meynell, Paul, "The Role of Lipids," *Your Start,* Neo-Life Company of America, 1978, p. C-73-4.

BOTHERED BY A BLOATED BELLY?

[1] Alsleben, H. Rudolph and Wilfrid Shute, *How to Survive the New Health Catastrophes,* Survivial Publications, Inc., 1973, p. 3-41.
[2] Clark, Linda, "Enzymes Can Help Your Health," *Let's Live,* June 1977, p. 62.

3 Alsleben, Rudolph, *How to Survive the New Health Catastrophes*, p. 3-41.

4 Clark, Linda, *Secrets of Health and Beauty*, Pyramid Books, 1975, p. 46.

Alsleben, Rudolph, *How to Survive the New Health Catastrophes*, p. 3-40.

6 Philpott, William H., "Proteolytic Enzyme and Amino Acid Therapy in Degenerative Disease," *A Physician's Handbook on Orthomolecular Medicine*, edited by Roger J. Williams and Dwight K. Kalita, Pergamon Press, 1977, pp. 1-2.

7 Clark, Linda, *Secrets of Health and Beauty*, p. 46.

8 Yudkin, John, "Sugar and Disease," *Nature*, Vol. 239, September 22, 1972, p. 198.

9 Prevention Magazine Staff, ed., *The Encyclopedia of Common Diseases*, Rodale Press, Inc., 1976, p. 1117.

10 Philpott, William, "Proteolytic Enzyme and Amino Acid Therapy in Degenerative Disease," p. 2.

11 Pritikin, Nathan, Jon Leonard and J.L. Hofer, *Live Longer Now*, Grosset and Dunlap, 1977, p. 51.

12 Alsleben, Rudolph, *How to Survive the New Health Catastrophes*, p. 3-41.

13 Clark, Linda, *Secrets of Health and Beauty*, p. 43.

14 Alsleben, Rudolph, *How to Survive the New Health Catastrophes*, pp. 3-41-2.

15 Tuckey, E. Hugh, "The Human Need for Hydrochloric Acid," *National Health Federation Bulletin*, October 1967, pp. 14-15.

16 *Ibid.*, p. 15.

17 Alsleben, Rudolph, *How to Survive the New Health Catastrophes, p. 3-42.*

18 Tuckey, E. Hugh, "The Human Need for Hydrochloric Acid," p. 15.

19 *Ibid., loc. cit.*

20 Clark, Linda, *Secrets of Health and Beauty*, p. 47.

21 Tuckey, E. Hugh, "The Human Need for Hydrochloric Acid," pp. 16-17.

22 Philpott, William, "Proteolytic Enzyme and Amino Acid Therapy in Degenerative Disease," p. 3.

23 Tuckey, E. Hugh, "The Human Need for Hydrochloric Acid," p. 17.

24 Long, James W., *The Essential Guide to Prescription Drugs*, Harper and Row, 1977, pp. 102-106.

25 Tuckey, E. Hugh, "The Human Need for Hydrochloric Acid," p. 17.

26 Clark, Linda, *Secrets of Health and Beauty*, p. 58.

[27] Rodale, J.I. and Staff, ed., *Best Health Articles from Prevention,* Rodale Books, Inc., 1967, p. 713.

[28] *Ibid., p. 711.*

[29] Clark, Linda, *Enzymes Can Help Your Health,* pp. 56-57.

[30] *Ibid.,* p. 58.

[31] Philpott, William, "Proteolytic Enzyme and Amino Acid Therapy in Degenerative Disease," p. 1.

[32] Ibid., p. 2.

[33] *Ibid.,* p. 3-4.

[34] *Ibid.,* p. 6.

[35] *Ibid.,* p. 7.

[36] Fredericks, Carlton and Herman Goodman, *Low Blood Sugar and You,* Grosset and Dunlap, c. 1969, p. 67.

[37] Shute, Wilfrid and Harald Taub, *Vitamin E for Ailing and Healthy Hearts,* Pyramid House, 1969, pp. 143-150.

[38] Pritikin, Nathan, *Live Longer Now,* p. 51.

[39] *Ibid.,* p. 8.

[40] Clark, Linda, "Enzymes Can Help Your Health," p. 62.

[41] Philpott, William, "Proteolytic Enzyme and Amino Acid Therapy in Degenerative Disease," p. 3.

TOOTH DECAY — SCOURGE OF THE CIVILIZED WORLD

[1] Weir, C. Edith, *Benefits from Human Nutrition Research,* U.S. Department of Agriculture, 1971, p. 64.

[2] Williams, Roger, *Nutrition Against Disease,* Bantam, 1973, p. 118.

[3] *Ibid.,* p. 119.

[4] Yudkin, John, "Sugar and Disease", *Nature,* September 22, 1972, p. 197.

[5] Williams, p. 123.

[6] Yudkin, John, "Sugar and Disease", *Nature,* September 22, 1972, pp. 197-199.

[7] McCormick, Paul M., "The Legal, Ethical and Political Implications of Fluoridation", *Cancer Control Journal,* Vol. 5, No. 1 & 2, pp. 84-85.

[8] Lee, John R., "Optimal Fluoridation", *The Western Journal of Medicine,* May 1975, p. 432.

[9] *Ibid.,* pp. 431-436.

[10] *Cancer Control Journal,* p. 142.

[11] Jerard, Elise, and J. B. Patrick, "The Summing of Fluoride Exposures", *International Journal of Environmental Studies,*

1973, Vol. 4, pp. 141-155.
12 Schatz, Albert and Vivian Schatz, "Use of Compost Instead of Chemical Fertilizer to Avoid Fluorine Contamination of Soil, Water, and Food", *Cancer Control Journal,* Vol. 5, No. 1 & 2, p. 145.
13 Burgstahler, Albert W., "Brief Report on Water Fluoridation", *National Fluoridation News,* October-December 1977, p. 4.
14 Schatz, Albert, "Increased Death Rates in Chile Associated with Artificial Fluoridation of Drinking Water, with Implications for Other Countries", *Journal of Arts, Science and Humanities,* Anthony University, January, 1976.
15 "Fluorides in Water may be Genetic Hazard", *Chemical and Engineering News,* September 20, 1976.
16 Massler, Maury and Issaac Schour, "Relation of Endemic Dental Fluorosis to Malnutrition", *Journal of the American Dental Association,* February 1952, pp. 163-164.
17 "Air Pollution Could Cause Mankind to Starve", *Cancer Control Journal,* Vol. 5, No. 1 & 2, p. 134.
18 "Fluoride Industry's Phantom Air Pollutant — Poisoning Animals, Farm and Forest", *Cancer Control Journal,* Vol. 5, No. 1 & 2, pp. 120ff.
19 *Ibid.,* p. 136.
20 *Ibid,* p. 165.
21 Mayron, Lewis, John Ott, Edward Amontree, and Rick Nations, "Light, Radiation, and Dental Caries", *Academic Therapy,* Vol. X, No. 4, Summer 1975, p. 441.
22 *Ibid.,* pp. 446-447.
23 *Ibid., loc. cit.*

NUTRITION AND SOCIAL PROBLEMS

1 McCarrison, Sir Robert and H.M. Sinclair, *Nutrition and Health,* Faber and Faber Limited, 1953, pp. 29-30.
2 Pottenger, Francis M., "The Effect of Heat Processed Foods and Metabolized Vitamin D Milk on the Dentofacial Structures of Experimental Animals," *American Journal of Orthodontics and Oral Surgery,* August 1946, p. 469.
3 Williams, Roger, *Nutrition Against Disease,* Bantam Books, 1973, p. 43.
4 Cheraskin, Dr. E.; W.M. Ringsdorf Jr.; and Arline Brecher, *Psychodietetics,* 1976, p. 88.
5 *Ibid.,* p. 89.

[6] "Zinc Deficiency May Cause Abnormal Aggressiveness," *San Francisco Chronicle*, October 6, 1975, p. 39.

[7] Pfeiffer, Carl C., *Mental and Elemental Nutrients*, Keats Publishin, Inc., 1975, p. 227.

[8] *Ibid.*, p. 230.

[9] Price, Weston, *Nutrition and Physical Degeneration*, Price-Pottenger Nutrition Foundation, 1975, p. 353.

[10] *Ibid.*, p. 354.

[11] *Ibid.*, p. 355.

[12] Libby, Alfred F., and Irwin Stone, "The Hypoascorbemia-Kwashiorkor Approach to Drug Addiction Therapy: A Pilot Study," *Journal of Orthomolecular Psychiatry*, Vol. 6, Fourth Quarter of 1977, No. 4, p. 300.

[13] *Ibid.*, pp. 301-303.

[14] "Enlist in the War Against Alcohol," Southern Publishing Association, 1978, p. 11.

[15] *Ibid., loc. cit.*

[16] Williams, Roger, *Nutrition Against Disease*, p. 177.

[17] "Enlist in the War Against Alcohol," p. 17.

[18] *Ibid.*, p. 14.

[19] McClintic, J. Robert, *Physiology of the Human Body*, John Wiley and Sons, 1975, p. 485.

[20] *Ibid.*, pp. 482-484.

[21] *Ibid.*, p. 486.

[22] Pfeiffer, Carl, *Mental and Elemental Nutrients*, p. 229.

[23] *Ibid.*, p. 225.

[24] *Ibid., loc. cit.*

[25] Long, James W., *Prescription Drugs*, Harper and Row, 1977, p. 282.

[26] Yudkin, John, *Sweet and Dangerous*, Bantam Books, 1973, p. 152.

[27] Ott, John Nash, *Health and Light*, Pocket Books, 1976, p. 53.

[28] Peters, R.R.; L.T. Chapin, K.B. Leining, and H.A. Tucker, "Supplemental Lighting Stimulates Growth and Lactation in Cattle," *Newsletter of the Center for Light Research*, Vol. 7, No. 1 1978, p. 4.

[29] "Do You Want to Lose the Hair on Your Chest?" Lee Foundation for Nutritional Research, Reprint No. 59.

IMPORTANCE OF IMPROVING THE AMERICAN DIET

[1] Rodale, J.I. and Staff, "Health in the Sea?", *Best Health Articles*

from Prevention Magazine, Rodale Press, 1967, p. 517.
2 *Ibid., loc. cit.*
3 Pfeiffer, Carl C., *Mental and Elemental Nutrients*, Keats Publishing, Inc., 1975, p. 3-4.
4 Williams, Roger J., *Nutrition Against Disease*, Bantam Books, 1973, p. 104.
5 *Ibid.*, p. 103-104.
6 Mickey, Karl B., *Health From the Ground Up*, International Harvester Company, 1946, p. 106.
7 Schubert, Bruno H., *Survival of Mankind*, Free-Economy Association, Inc., 1967, p. 39.
8 Lappe, Frances Moore, *Diet for a Small Planet*, Ballantine, 1975, p. 31.
9 Mickey, Karl B., *Health From the Ground Up*, p. 68.
10 *Ibid., loc. cit.*
11 Elwood, Catharyn, *Feel Like a Million*, Pocket Books, 1956, p. 19.
12 Schubert, Bruno H., *Survival of Mankind*, p. 29, 30, 39.
13 Seroy, William W., "Chelated Minerals - A Key to Better Health", National Health Federation Bulletin, January, 1972, p. 22-23.
14 Chase, Alice, *Nutrition for Health*, Parker Publishing Co., Inc., 1970, p. 240.
15 Alsleben, Rudolph, *How to Survive the New Health Catastrophes*, p. 9.
16 Schubert, Bruno H., *Survival of Mankind*, p. 9.
17 *Ibid.*, p. 31.
18 Yudkin, John, "Sugar and Disease", *Nature*, September 22, 1972, p. 197.
19 *Ibid.*, p. 197-200.
20 Fredericks, Carlton, "Hotline to Health", *Prevention Magazine* January 1975, p. 47-48.
21 Jacobson, Michael F., *Eater's Digest*, Doubleday Anchor, 1972, p. 4-10.
22 Williams, Roger J., *Nutrition Against Disease*, p. 64.
23 Jacobson, Michael F., *Eater's Digest*, p. 36.
24 *"Summary-Review"*, Mineral Lab, Inc., p. 5-8.
25 Cheraskin, E., Ringsdorf, W.M. and Clark, J.w., *Diet and Disease* Keats Publishing, Inc., 1968, p. 15-16.
26 Williams, Roger J., *Nutrition Against Disease*, p. 27.
27 *Ibid.*, p. 27.
28 *Ibid.*, p. 52.
29 Ibid., loc. cit.
30 *Ibid.*, p. 59.
31 "Brain Cells — Cheap", *The Globe and Mail*, July 4, 1972.
32 Williams, Roger J., *Nutrition Against Disease*, p. 19.

33 *Ibid.*, p. 24.
34 *Ibid.*, p. 138.

MEDICINE IN THE 21st CENTURY

1 "Index of Nutritional Abnormalities Induced by 50 Commonly Prescribed Drugs," IMA Publications Division: La Jolla, Calif. 1978.
2 Illiych, Ivan, *Medical Nemesis,* Bantam Books, 1977, p. 17.
3 *Ibid.*, p. 66.
4 *Ibid.*, p. 65.
5 *Ibid., p. 19*
6 *Ibid., loc. cit.*
7 Long, James W., *The Essential Guide to Prescription Drugs,* Harper and Row, 1977, pp. 366-7.
8 *Ibid.*, p. 473.
9 *Ibid.*, p. 703.
10 Rodale, J. I., *Best Health Articles from Prevention,* Rodale Books, 1967, p. 208.
11 Illiych, *Medical Nemesis,* p. 22.
12 *Ibid.*, p. 23.
13 Williams, Roger Jr., *Nutrition Against Disease,* Pitman Publishing Corporation, 1971, p. 8.
14 *Ibid.*, p. 3.
15 Livingston, Virginia, *Cancer: A New Breakthrough,* Production House Publishers, 1972, p. 108.
16 Kalita, Dwight K., and Williams, Roger J., *A Physician's Handbook on Orthomolecular Medicine,* Pergamon Press, 1977, p. 152.
17 McKeown, Thomas, "Determinants of Health," *Human Nature,* April 1978, pp. 62-3.
18 *Ibid.*, p. 64.
19 Williams, Roger J., *Biochemical Individuality,* University of Texas Press, 1975, pp. 166-176.
20 *Ibid.*, p. 15.
21 Williams, *Nutrition Against Disease,* p. 25.
22 *Ibid.*, p. p. 53.
23 Bieler, Henry, *Food is Your Best Medicine,* Vintage Books, 1973, p. 42.
24 *Ibid., p. 41-2.*
25 *Ibid.*, p. 40.
26 Alsleben, H. Rudolph, *How to Survive the New Health Catastrophes,* Survival Publications, 1973, p. 3-51.

27 Shelton, Herbert M., *Fasting for Renewal of Life*, Natural Hygiene Press, 1974, p. 215.

28 Cheraskin, E., Ringsdorf, W. M., and Clark, J. W., *Diet and Disease*, Keats Publishing, Inc., 1977, p. 90-91.

29 Yudkin, John, "Sugar and Disease", *Nature*, vol. 239, September 22, 1972, pp. 197-199. (See also: Cheraskin, E., Ringsdorf, W. M. and Ramsay, R. R., "Sucrose, neutrophilic phagocytosis and resistance to disease," *Dental Survey*, December 1976, p. 46.)

30 Leonard, Jon N., Hofer, J. L., and Pritikin, N., *Live Longer Now*, Grosset and Dunlap, 1977, pp. 26-7.

31 *Ibid.*, pp. 75-6.

32 Alsleben, *Health Catastrophes*, p. 3-41.

33 Williams, *Nutrition Against Disease*, p. 47.

34 Kalita, *Physician's Handbook*, p. 5.

35 Williams, *Nutrition Against Disease*, p. 25.

36 Williams, Roger J., *You Are Extraordinary*, Pyramid Books, 1976, p. 27.

37 *Ibid.*, p. 54.

38 *Ibid.*, p. 63.

39 Clark, Linda, *Stay Young Longer*, Pyramid Books, 1977, p. 29.

40 Cheraskin, E., and Ringsdorf, W. M., *Predictive Medicine*, Pacific Press Publishing Association, 1973, p. 45.

41 *Ibid.*, p. 49.

42 Kalita, *Physician's Handbook*, p. 148.

INDEX

FOR ADDITIONAL INFORMATION

For information about other "Image" Awareness publications, lectures, seminars, tapes, or additional copies of this book contact the "Image" Awareness Corporation, P.O. Box 3307, Auburn, California 95604.

For information concerning the photographs used in this book and other excellent material on different aspects of nutrition, contact the Price-Pottenger Nutrition Foundation, P.O. Box 2614, La Mesa, California 92041.

Power To Live Through Nutrition is available at a 30% discount for orders of 10 or more books.

Quantity	Total
________ Books @ $6.95	$ ________
Less 30% discount for orders of 10 or more	$ ________
Total for books	$ ________
California residents add 6% tax	$ ________
Postage & handling 50¢ per book	$ ________
Total enclosed	$ ________

Ship to ____________________

Street address ____________________

City ____________ State ________ Zip ____________

Mail to:
Image Awareness Corporation
P.O. Box 3307
Auburn, CA 95604